DOWN AND DIRTY
SEX SECRETS

ALSO BY TRISTAN TAORMINO

The Ultimate Guide to Anal Sex for Women

Previously published under the title
Pucker Up

ReganBooks
An Imprint of HarperCollins*Publishers*

DOWN ᴬⁿᵈ DIRTY
SEX SECRETS

THE NEW AND NAUGHTY GUIDE
TO BEING GREAT IN BED

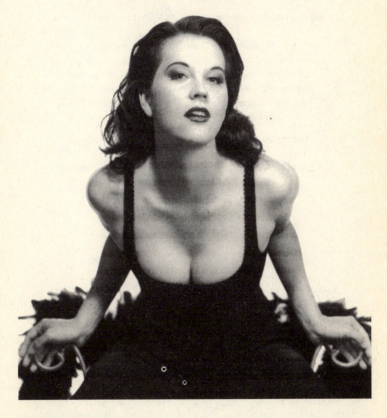

TRISTAN TAORMINO

A hardcover edition of this book was published in 2001
by ReganBooks, an imprint of HarperCollins Publishers,
under the title *Pucker Up.*

Cover and title page photograph by Richard Mitchell
Hair and makeup by Tatijana Suljic-Shoan

All illustrations © 2000 by Fish. The illustration "Female Anatomy,
Front View" first appeared in *The Clitoral Truth: The Secret World at
Your Fingertips* by Rebecca Chalker (New York: Seven Stories Press,
2000). The illustrations "Female Anatomy, Side View,"
"Male Anatomy," and "Anorectal Anatomy" first appeared in
The Ultimate Guide to Anal Sex for Women by Tristan Taormino
(San Francisco: Cleis Press, 1997).

HarperCollins books may be purchased for educational,
business, or sales promotional use.
For information please write: Special Markets Department,
HarperCollins Publishers Inc.,
10 East 53rd Street, New York, NY 10022.

First paperback edition published 2003.

Designed by Katharine Nichols

The Library of Congress has cataloged the
hardcover edition under its original title as follows:

Taormino, Tristan, 1971–
Pucker up: a hands-on guide to ecstatic sex / Tristan Taormino.
—1st ed.
p. cm.
ISBN 0-06-039415-3
    1. Sex instruction for women. 2. Sex instruction for men. I. Title.
HQ46 .T237 2001
613.9'6—dc21

2001277580

ISBN 0-06-098892-4 (pbk.)

   03   04   05   06   07   RRD   10   9   8   7   6   5   4   3   2

for Red

Contents

Acknowledgments

I am so thankful to my original editor, Tia Maggini, who worked her butt off on the book; her diligent readings of the manuscript and insightful suggestions were invaluable to the final product. Publisher Judith Regan, senior editor Dana Albarella, and everyone at ReganBooks supported me with advice, ideas, and plenty of encouragement. Fish created the unique illustrations which bring my words to life, and I feel blessed to collaborate with such a talented artist again. Richard Mitchell worked his incredible magic when he took the inspired cover photo, and makeup artist Tatijana Suljic-Shoan made me glamorous. Kudos too to art director Ron de la Peña for his fabulous cover design. Thanks to my agent, Andrew Blauner, for all his hard work (and for Friday night phone calls!). He continues to be an unflinching advocate, champion, and friend to me, which I appreciate more than he probably knows.

I have learned something from every editor I have ever worked with, but, most recently, I owe a debt of gratitude to my editor at *The Village Voice*, Doug Simmons, whose guidance has deeply influenced my sex writing. Felice Newman, Frédérique Delacoste, Don Weise, and everyone at Cleis Press were there when it all began.

Claire Potter was a great teacher. There are dozens of sexperts and pioneers who've come before me and whose work has had a tremendous influence on my own, and some must be named: Kim Airs, Joani Blank, Susie Bright, Fairy Butch, Patrick Califia-Rice, Rebecca Chalker, Betty Dodson, Heather Findlay, Nina Hartley, Bert Herrman, Robert Lawrence, FetishDiva Midori, Jack Morin, Carol Queen, Anne Seamans, Annie Sprinkle, Debi Sundahl, and Cathy Winks. Gene Trent of Blue Door Video generously lent me countless adult videos to watch for this book and never complained when I returned them late.

Rachel Kramer Bussel has contributed her time, energy, hard work, friendship, and wonderful spirit to me and to this project, especially in pulling together the Resource Guide. All the babes (past, present, and future) of Toys in Babeland (especially Alicia, Rachel, and Tova) inspire me with their enthusiasm and dedication to improving the sex lives of people everywhere. Owner Claire Cavanah gave me the best job in the world and lavishes unbelievable amounts of support on me. My gratitude to all the sex-toy-store owners who have hosted my workshops, and everyone who attended them, especially those brave enough to ask me a question. Thanks to my fans (you know who you are)—you keep me up when I am down.

Without the support of the people closest to me, I couldn't do any of it. My assistant, Michelle Cronk, makes it all happen smoothly. Jill, Marisa, and Dr. Y keep me healthy. My family and friends love me, listen to me, and spoil me: Toni Amato (the best big brother in the world), Morgan Dunbar (since the very beginning), Mario Grillo (God bless America), Sarah Jones (an expert in many fields), Stan Kent (guardian angel), Ira Levine (kindred perverted spirit), Audrey Prins-Patt (queen of the clitoris), Winston Wilde (daddy and sexologist rolled into one), Mom and Dad (who got me here). Mom and Rachel, thanks for help with the title.

And finally to Red, my partner, my love. You are in this book on every page, and more important, in my heart always.

DOWN AND DIRTY SEX SECRETS

Introduction

The Joy of Fucking

I peddled dildos for a living, and it changed my life. As a salesperson at the women-owned sex-toy shop Toys in Babeland in New York City, I actually sold more than rubber dongs and silicone cocks. The shelves are filled with products designed for pleasure—vibrators, lubricants, condoms, butt plugs, massage oils, leather harnesses, paddles, anal beads, blindfolds, nipple clamps, latex gloves, and adult videos. But the store offers something else that is perhaps more valuable than even the most expensive toys: honest, useful information and advice about sexuality.

Every day I worked there, dozens of ordinary folks walked through the door looking for what we had inside. Their searches almost always began with a question. Most of them were complete strangers, and yet they told me things about themselves that were extremely personal and deeply intimate. Their revelations were sometimes moving, sometimes surprising, and always fascinating.

A been-there-done-that rocker chick strutted toward me one day, all pierced and tattooed, and I was sure she was headed for the S/M section at the back of the store; instead, she said, "I'm here to buy my first vibrator." A middle-aged stockbroker, who looked out of place next to a table of colorful anal toys, took an hour to summon the nerve to tell me he wanted a penis pump and a book on tantric sex. A city bus driver, still in uniform and just off work, came in with his wife; they meandered around the store, speaking in whispers to each other, then approached me. She looked at her feet shyly, and he did all the talking. They wanted a strap-on dildo for her to do him in the ass. I figured out pretty quickly that I could never assume anything about anyone's sex life by simply looking at the person.

I also learned to be as neutral and objective as possible when hearing people's concerns, queries, and individual situations. I needed to listen without bias or judgment. I needed to leave behind my own sexual preferences and preoccupations in order to meet my customers where they stood at the moment. Across boundaries of race, class, gender, sexual orientation, age, ability, and education, I had to listen and respond to some very important issues, problems, and desires. I usually left work feeling less like a retail clerk and more like a sex therapist.

Feeling like a sex therapist was somewhat familiar to me. After my first book, *The Ultimate Guide to Anal Sex for Women,* was published in 1998, I needed a unique way to promote it. As you can imagine, it did not exactly lend itself to the traditional book reading. Most bookstores weren't clamoring to create a huge poster of the cover, put it in the window, and announce a book signing by me. It was no *Chicken Soup for Your Ass,* even if I thought it was. Distributors were concerned that people would be too embarrassed to even buy it because of its taboo topic. It was only the second book ever devoted to this particular sexual subject, and I believed it was an important and necessary one. I wanted so much to spread the word about the ecstatic possibilities of anal sex. I decided to embark on a mission to teach the world how to have safe and pleasurable anal sex; in the process, if I sold some books, that would be a bonus. I traveled around the country teaching workshops in order to replace some of the myths and misconceptions about this forbidden act with facts and specific information.

My workshops were an opportunity to talk about sex in an honest, straightforward, down-to-earth way. For some of my students, an anal-sex class was their first opportunity to have a frank discussion about *anything* sexual. For others, it was a chance to be in a room full of like-minded people who validated their own desires, desires they may have kept hidden for a long time. Some even told me that it had been a life-affirming and life-changing event. Empowering people to get in touch with their asses—and their sexuality in general—was my goal. But in the process of teaching, I found that I was learning not just about the sex lives of individuals, but about the state of sex in our culture.

I believe that sex is one of the most important aspects of our lives, but our society does not treat it as such. Sexuality is still trivialized, marginalized, and denigrated by most of our cultural institutions (including science and religion) or exploited and oversimplified by others, like the media. So many of us are taught to emphasize the important things in life—our partners, our children, our families, our careers, our spirituality, and our health. Once we've taken care of all these aspects, then we have permission to think about sex, which is seen as less worthy than most everything else.

But sex is a significant part of us, one that is rich with opportunities to learn, explore, connect, heal, and grow. Sex is a way to express ourselves and to communicate with others—a chance to create a unique, intimate bond with another human being.

My passion for understanding and celebrating sex has fueled the writing of this book. And so has each and every person who's had the courage to ask me a question about sex. Teaching sex workshops and working at Toys in Babeland has given me so much insight into what is going on in the minds and bedrooms of people across America. My work has given me a vision of what kinds of things people are interested in, what elements of sexuality spark the most questions, what subjects there is clearly not enough information about, what excites people, what shocks them, what turns them on.

Through my sex-education career, I have also discovered upcoming trends for sex. These activities aren't newly discovered or invented, but rather they are a new part of public consciousness. Most of them have been around for a long time, but have not captured the interest of sex researchers or the imagination of everyday people. In this new century, sex and relationships are rapidly changing. We are poised to enter an entirely new realm of sexuality, where old taboos are busted and more and more people are open to bold, expansive ideas about sex. At this moment in history, so many things once considered alternative or on the fringe—whether lesbian and gay sexuality, S/M, tantric sex, or open sexual relationships—are becoming more popular and gaining more mainstream acceptance. People's dirty little secrets don't seem that dirty anymore, and what was once forbidden has just moved in with the girl next door. A new revolution is in order, and as *The Joy of Sex* was part of the sexual revolution of the 1970s, so I offer my new guide: I like to think of it as *The Joy of Fucking*.

Whenever I tell people what I do, whether I say I wrote a book on anal sex, worked at a sex-toy store, or write a sex column, they almost always have a question for me. A question they've been carrying around, one they haven't been able to ask a lover, a friend, a parent, or a doctor. As diverse, unique, and meaningful as the people who ask them, all these questions formed the basis of this book. They span different sexual identities, experiences, preferences, and points of view. But in the end, we are all more similar than different when it comes to sex. Most of us want to know as much as we can about our sexuality and that of our partners in order to have the very best sex we can. This book is my way of answering all the questions I've ever been asked. Whenever someone asks a question at a public event, inevitably, I see nods of recognition and looks of curiosity around the room. A great question is one that many people want the answer to, and I hope that the responses in this book will benefit more than just the people who first inquired.

I begin with a chapter on anatomy and orgasm; think of it as the instruction manual they forgot to include with our bodies. In this section, I also explore new ideas about the clitoris being not just one structure but an entire system, which may make you rethink your ideas about female sexual anatomy. In chapter 2, I move beyond the body to the heart and mind to delve into the intricate territory of desire. How do we find out what turns us on? Once we know, then what do we do about it? I cover sexual communication, from the simple to the saucy, in the hopes that I may get you talking more about sex. Improving your sexual communication skills (and your partner's) brings you one step closer to getting your needs and desires fulfilled. Talking about safer sex, and how to incorporate it into your relationship, is also in this chapter. You'll find tips and techniques on refining your hand-job and oral-sex skills in chapter 3.

The fourth chapter puts you smack dab in the middle of a sex-toy store; this is my virtual tour of a variety of pleasure products. I highlight different kinds of lubricants and how they can enhance all sexual activities. I take you through buying your first vibrator, using it alone or with a partner, and I include styles, popular brands, and tried and true techniques. Likewise, we'll explore the delicious world of dildos—the different kinds and the ins and outs of using them. In chapter 5, I offer a wide range of information and insight about G-spot stimulation, from anatomical directions and position ideas to G-spot toys and tricks. In addition, I introduce you to a long-misunderstood phenomenon: female ejaculation. You'll learn about the history of female ejaculation, what it is, and how to make yourself or your partner ejaculate.

Everything you ever wanted to know about anal pleasure for both men and women is in chapter 6. Look for some myths to be replaced with truths and plenty of information about one of my favorite subjects. I'll give you tips on preparation and positions, tools and techniques, G-spot and prostate stimulation, and strap-on sex. Being able to share your fantasies with a lover is such an important component to a great sexual relationship. In chapter 7, learn how to tap into your own and your partner's fantasies, share them with each other, and even fulfill some of them. The orchestration of role playing—including the who, what, when, where, and why, with plenty of examples—will help you create your own sexy erotic dramas.

Following fantasy, in chapter 8, we move on to the numerous ways in which you can incorporate erotica, including magazines, books, and adult videos, into your sex life for stimulation, inspiration, and exploration. Chapter 9 is dedicated to BDSM: the pleasures of pain, the power of dominance and submission, and more. Learn how to determine if you're a top or a bottom and how to negotiate and execute a scene. Dive into a world of bondage, sensory deprivation, spanking, flogging, hot wax, psychological play, and even wilder activities.

In all nine chapters, I have highlighted one specific question and answer that relates to the subject of the chapter. They are actual questions selected from the hundreds people have asked me on the job and thousands of letters and e-mails. Throughout the book I will refer you to other sources where you can get further information about some of the practices, products, and ideas I discuss. At the end of the book, I offer a very extensive Resource Guide—full of books, video titles and producers, sex-toy stores, catalogs, BDSM companies, hot lines, Web sites, and sexuality workshops—to guide you in the right direction.

From "How to Drive Your Woman Wild in Bed" at the Learning Annex to "How to Female Ejaculate" at The Michigan Womyn's Music Festival, I have taught more than one hundred sex workshops around the country full of information people can really use. I wrote this book to respond to popular questions and give honest, useful information that doesn't shy away from sensitive topics. Extraordinary sex doesn't just happen; it takes dedication and hard work. In other words, you need to make it happen. Hopefully, there are some tools in this book that will help you achieve your personal goals. And speaking of goals, there is enough pressure in our society to be superwoman or superman and be perfect in everything we do. That is not what this book is about.

This book is my gift to all its readers, a chance for me to share my knowledge about sex with you. When two people come together sexually, they make a deal, whether spoken or symbolic, to take a trip together. When you are involved in an emotional relationship with a sexual partner and you know that person well, you develop a closeness and a trust. Your relationship is the perfect setting to challenge each other, explore your boundaries, become adventurous, and see where sex can take you. I want to give you the tools you need to get wherever you are going.

REDEFINING EROGENOUS ZONES AND ORGASM

Sexual Anatomy and Response

The Anatomy Lesson

I always begin my sex workshops with an anatomy lesson. I don't want to bore my students or give them flashbacks to high school biology class, but I can't assume that everyone has detailed knowledge about physiology. You would be amazed at how little most people know about their own sexual anatomy! Most of us weren't paying close attention to that particular lecture in health class, and many people, sadly, have never looked closely at their own genitals. There is a reason that feminists in the 1970s were whipping out those plastic speculums and hand-held mirrors at consciousness-raising groups all over the country. When women and men have a better understanding of our bodies, we feel less alienated from them. Knowledge is the first step toward being more in tune with your body.

From the important anatomical structures and where they are located to their different functions and how they may contribute to pleasure and orgasm, knowing more about your own body and how it works can give you a better grasp of how you experience sexual pleasure. Of course, sex is not just physical; emotional, psychological, and spiritual aspects of eroticism are just as important as our working parts. I don't want to diminish their significance in any way; however, it's crucial for people to get better acquainted with their bodies and those of their partners if they want to give them boundless pleasure.

When I began research for my book *The Ultimate Guide to Anal Sex for Women*, I wanted to gather as much information as possible about anorectal anatomy. Since my background was in sexual activism and writing, the scientific and medical aspects of anal sex were less familiar to me. Naively, I thought that anatomy—including our sexual anatomy—was a science based on "hard facts." You know, anatomists cut open a cadaver and sketched out all the organs. Then, they hooked some live people up to machines, monitored how different anatomical structures functioned, and took lots of notes. I believed that everyone at least agreed on where everything was located. Was I in for a big shock.

What I discovered is that, like the social sciences, anatomy is open to different interpretations and schools of thought. And when it comes to sexual anatomy, particularly women's sexual anatomy, we girls have been given the short end of the information stick. First, it seems that anatomists know each minute detail of every millimeter of the penis, but they do not have comparable detailed information about the vulva, the clitoris, or the G-spot. In fact, the lack of information about female sexual anatomy and function is startling. Second, many anatomical drawings and explanations are often vague when it comes to the intricacies of female genitalia; these texts either gloss over or disregard altogether entire structures that are important to our sexual anatomy. When depictions and descriptions do reference particular parts, they fail to explain their function, their relationship to other structures, or their role in sexual arousal and orgasm. This lack of information leaves us in the dark about our bodies and maintains the "mystery" of female genitalia for both women and men.

As a result of misinformation (and a lack of *any* information in some cases), feminist doctors, scientists, sexologists, health-care advocates, and activists decided to do their own research. Two particular groups produced significant research that has become the cornerstone of a new school of thought about the female body. The Boston Women's Health Collective published the first edition of *Our Bodies, Ourselves* in 1969, and it has produced several subsequent revised editions of *The New Our Bodies, Ourselves* (the most recent was released in 1998). While the book was not specifically about sex, *Our Bodies, Ourselves* contributed greatly to women's understanding of their sexuality. The first time I heard the word "clitoris," I went straight to the index of this classic to see what everyone was talking about!

The Federation of Feminist Women's Health Centers (FFWHCs), an organization of women's health clinics around the country, published a groundbreaking book called *A New View of a Woman's Body: An Illustrated Guide* in 1981. Written by the women of FFWHCs, this insightful book offered us a completely revised perspective on female sexual anatomy with a specific focus on the clitoris. What the writers of the book (and certainly plenty of feminists) saw as the most egregious error in the male-centered view of sexual anatomy was the focus on the vagina as the primary female sexual organ—the one most comparable to the penis. This book argued a different point of view: the *clitoris* is most anatomically analogous to the penis, and, more importantly, it is much more crucial to women's sexual pleasure than the vagina. In addition to identifying the clitoris as the center of our sexual universe, the FFWHCs wanted to expand its anatomical reach as well.

The authors of *A New View* blasted the mainstream concept of the clitoris being only a small nub of sensitive flesh protected by a hood above the vaginal opening. Instead, they recast the clitoris to encompass not just the clitoral glans and shaft (the nub), but also the inner lips, the frenulum, the vaginal opening, the urethra and urethral sponge. Shifting our entire understanding of female sexuality, feminists hoped to empower women with this new conceptualization of their bodies. Most feminist sex educators, myself included, base our own work on this updated definition of women's anatomy and the far-reaching potential of the clitoris. Slowly, feminist efforts to expand the definition of the clitoris have seeped into mainstream medicine. For example, in a recent *Newsweek* article on female desire, John Leland told a revealing story: "In a conference room at Boston University, [Professor] Trudy Van Houten stops an unsuspecting medical student. *The clitoris,* she challenges the young woman, a fourth-year med student: *how big is it?* The woman looks momentarily stunned. *Would you say it's one centimeter or 10?* By the fourth year of medical school, students should know the gross details of the body, but this seemingly simple question has the woman in a pickle. 'It can't be as big as 10,' she tries. Oh, but it is, it is. 'It's here, it's here, it's here, it's here,' says Van Houten, tracing a finger across an anatomical drawing. 'Wow,' says the student."[1]

In 2000, Rebecca Chalker, the editor of *A New View of a Woman's Body,* published *The Clitoral Truth,* which took up where *A New View* left off, providing further information about women's genital anatomy and sexual pleasure, including expanded information on the clitoris and the G-spot.

Female Sexual Anatomy

The traditional definition of the vulva is the pubic mound, the outer and inner lips of the labia, the vaginal and urethral openings, and most of what is visible of the female genitals. In the newer understanding of women's sexual anatomy, the vulva consists of the pubic mound and the outer lips, which contain nerve endings but are nowhere near as rich in receptors as other parts of female sexual anatomy. The pubic mound and outer lips are formed from the same fetal tissue as the scrotal sac in men. Nearly every other structure in the area of the vagina—the inner lips, the frenulum, the clitoral glans and hood, the urethral opening, the urethral sponge, and the vaginal opening—is considered part of the clitoris. (See illustration 1.) This conclusion is based on the fact that these structures are comprised of the same fetal tissue as the penis glans and shaft, prostate gland, bulb, and related glands.[2]

Full of nerve endings, the inner lips surround the urethral opening, the urethral sponge, and the opening to the vagina and are more sensitive than the outer lips. Below the vaginal opening, as the lips come together, they form the fourchette, which signals the bottom boundary or end of the clitoris. They come to a point (called the frenulum) which forms the tissue of the clitoral hood. The hood protects the clitoral glans much like the foreskin of a penis.

Nestled inside the hood is the critical centerpiece of the clitoral system called the glans, an incredibly sensitive nub rich in nerve endings—an estimated six to eight thousand nerve endings make it *the* most sensitive spot on a human body. The glans is the external portion of (or end of) the clitoral shaft, a half-inch long structure composed of spongy erectile tissue. The clitoral glans is what traditional anatomists call the entire clitoris. Because of its abundance of nerve endings, the glans is hyper-responsive to all kinds of stimulation including stroking, rubbing, licking, and vibration. Beneath the layer of skin of the clitoris is a network of blood vessels, nerves, glands, muscles, and erectile tissue. During arousal, the erectile tissue fills with blood and becomes engorged and erect, a response which mirrors the male erection.

Below the clitoral glans and hood and above the vaginal opening is the opening to the urethra, a two-inch tube leading from the bladder to the urethral opening through which women urinate. (See illustration 2.) The urethra is surrounded

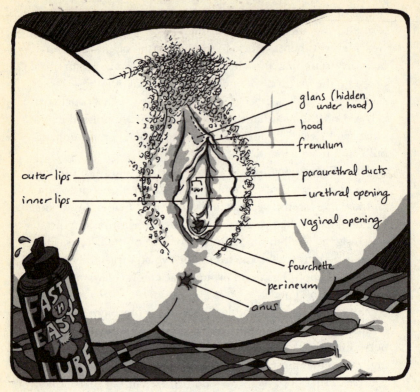

FIG. 1   FEMALE ANATOMY, FRONT VIEW

by the urethral sponge, also known to many as the G-spot. The spongy erectile tissue that makes up the urethral sponge contains paraurethral glands, which produce female ejaculatory fluid, a substance shown to be very similar to fluid produced by the prostate gland in men. When a woman is aroused, the erectile tissue of the sponge fills with blood and becomes erect, and the glands fill with fluid, all of which cause the urethral sponge to swell. Because it's more prominent when it swells, it is easier to locate when a woman is aroused; it is also very sensitive to pressure and stimulation. (Look for more information about the G-spot and female ejaculation in chapter 5.)

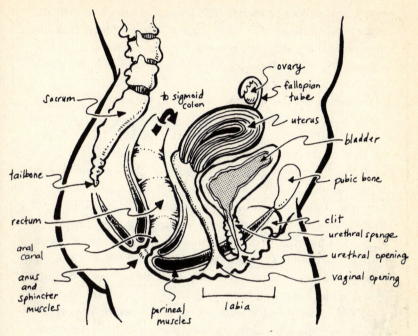

FIG. 2   FEMALE ANATOMY, SIDE VIEW

The opening to the vagina, located below the urethral opening, is muscular and contains a substantial amount of nerve endings (although nowhere near the amount of the clitoral glans). For most women, the vaginal opening and the lower portion of the vagina (including the G-spot on its front wall) are more sensitive than the rest of the vagina. Made up of elastic tissue, the vagina produces lubrication and its walls expand when a woman is aroused.

At the back of the vagina is the cervix, the opening to the uterus, through which menstrual blood flows. While it has no specific sexual function, it's a good idea to be aware of the cervix, especially during intercourse. In general, the cervix is very sensitive to any kind of strong pressure, and you can bruise or abrade it if you are not careful. If your partner has a particularly long penis or you are in a position that allows deep thrusting, chances are he will bump into it. Most women find this uncomfortable (although there are some women who like it) and need to tell their partners to change positions or the depth of penetration if necessary.

Women's genital anatomy is a complex system of nerves, blood vessels, glands, muscles, and tissue, with a variety of structures that connect, overlap, and work together. This new perspective of the clitoris encompassing the inner lips, the pelvic muscles, the clitoral glans and hood, and the urethral sponge brings us one step closer to comprehending female sexual response. Before the women's movement, popular notions of female sexual pleasure focused on the vagina as the perfect counterpart to the penis, and thus vaginal penetration as the source of a woman's orgasm. Some women who didn't come as a result of penetration alone felt as if there was something wrong with them. Feminists sought to "correct" the vaginally centered concept by focusing almost totally on the importance of clitoral stimulation, leaving some women who enjoyed penetration feeling their pleasure was discounted and discredited. Today, we have a much broader view of women's pleasure, which can be experienced through clitoral and G-spot stimulation, vaginal and anal stimulation, or any combination of activities.

Male Sexual Anatomy

I'll begin with the most obvious part of male sexual anatomy: the penis. The body of the penis is called the shaft and is comprised of spongy erectile tissue full of blood vessels. During arousal, the tissue fills with blood, the penis swells and becomes erect. The urethra, the tube through which men urinate, is located inside the shaft. (See illustration 3.)

The head of the penis, called the glans, is rich in nerve endings and is usually the most sensitive part of a man's sexual anatomy. At birth, the glans is surrounded and protected by a

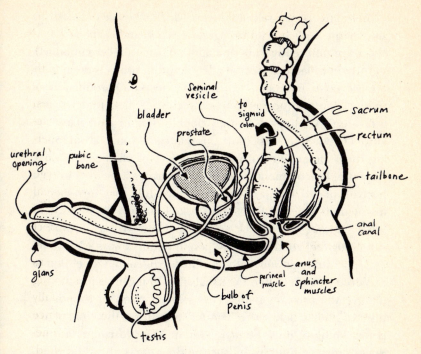

FIG. 3   MALE ANATOMY, SIDE VIEW

hood, the foreskin. When a penis is circumcised, this skin is cut off, leaving the glans mostly exposed. An uncircumcised penis has its foreskin intact; it surrounds and protects the glans much like the clitoral hood. Because it is "hidden" inside this sleeve of skin, an uncircumcised penis has a more sensitive glans than its circumcised brother. At the base of the glans is the coronal ridge, a sensitive spot which most men like stimulated. The urethral opening is also in the glans.

The base of the penis extends into a man's body, and the root (or bulb) of the penis can be felt through the perineum (which is between the anal opening and the testicles) or through the rectum. Many men find the bulb to be extremely sensitive to stimulation.

Below the penis are the testicles, which produce testosterone and sperm. Testicles can vary greatly in size and shape and may also hang differently from one another; they are contained in a sac of skin called the scrotum. The scrotum protects them from intense cold and heat, which can affect the production of sperm. Men tend to be quite protective of their testicles, and they aren't kidding when they double over in pain if they're kicked between the legs. Now, this may cause you to avoid touching them altogether during sex, for fear of eliciting the same response. I recommend you ask your partner if he likes to have his balls played with, and if he does, ask him for some specific instructions. Does he like them stroked, rubbed gently, tugged? Would he like you to lick and suck them? Will a little bit of stretching feel good to him? When in doubt, always ask.

Men are endowed with another erogenous zone that is explored less often than the usual spots, but can be just as stimulating: the prostate gland. The prostate gland surrounds the urethra and is below the bladder and above the root of the penis. Think of it as the male G-spot. The prostate gland produces prostatic fluid in the surrounding ducts; this fluid mixes with sperm in the vas deferens before a man ejaculates. Anal penetration is the best way to reach the prostate gland. You can stimulate it through the wall of the rectum if you go about three inches inside and aim toward his navel. Like a woman's G-spot, the prostate becomes more sensitive and receptive to stimulation when a man is aroused, so you should be nice and turned on before you explore any kind of prostate stimulation. The gland is very sensitive to massage, and most men prefer gentle rubbing; any jerky movement or poking can be very uncomfortable. Lots of men can have an orgasm from prostate stimulation without even touching their dicks! Always remember that each man's prostate gland is unique—some men may enjoy theirs stimulated and others may not. (For more on prostate stimulation, see chapter 6.)

Anal Anatomy

With the exception of the male prostate gland, men's and women's anal anatomy is nearly identical, so we share basically the same geography in this area of our bodies. (See illustration 4.)

Before you go anywhere near your back door, you need to meet its puckered front door, otherwise known as the anus. The external opening of the anal canal, the anus is rich in blood vessels and nerve endings which makes it incredibly receptive to touch, stimulation, and vibration. In fact, for some people, external stimulation of the anus is all they need to experience intense anal pleasure. The opening itself can be one of our most sensual erogenous zones.

In the tissue surrounding the anal opening are two sets of muscles: the anal sphincters. If you have ever penetrated someone anally with your finger, you know that just inside the anus, you feel a snug ring of muscle—those are the sphincter muscles. The external sphincter, which is closest to the opening, is controlled by the central nervous system, which also controls muscle movement. When you attempt to "hold on" to a bowel movement until you make it to the bathroom, you are using (and tensing) your external sphincter muscle. With patience and practice, you can learn to voluntarily control the external sphincter in other situations too, and make it relax instead of tense.

The internal sphincter is controlled by the autonomic nervous system, which controls involuntary bodily functions like your breathing rate. This muscle ordinarily reacts reflexively, and most people do not normally control its function; however, the external and the internal sphincters overlap and can work together. The rule of thumb is that the more attention you pay to the sphincters, the easier it is to relax them. Because the two muscles work in tandem, when one relaxes, the other does too.

Inside the anus and past the sphincter muscles is the anal canal, which is about one to one and a half inches long. The

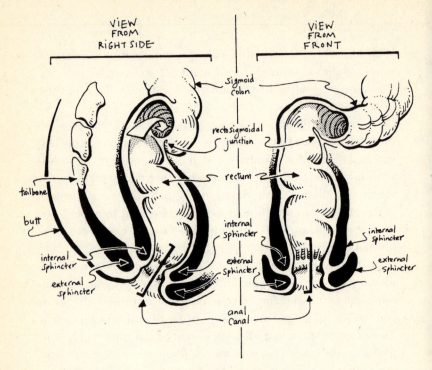

FIG. 4   ANAL ANATOMY

same soft, sensitive tissue that makes up the anus comprises the first portion of the anal canal, which is very sensitive to stimulation. The rest of the anal canal is composed of mucous membrane, also sensitive to touch, and more sensitive to pressure. Like the clitoris and penis, when you are aroused, the tissue of the anal canal fills with blood and becomes engorged. During arousal, when the muscles are relaxed, the anal canal has the ability to expand to make penetration very pleasurable.

Beyond the anal canal, the rectum occupies approximately the next eight inches. The rectum is made up of loose folds of soft, smooth tissue which is especially responsive to pressure and penetration. The rectum has a tremendous ability to expand and can be roomier than the anal canal—just think, during surgery, a doctor can put her entire hand in a person's rectum. The rectum is not a straight tube, but curves gently, which is crucial to know about before you put anything longer than a finger in someone else's butt or your own. The lower part of the rectum tilts slightly toward the navel for several inches, then curves back the other way toward the spine, then curves toward the navel again. These curves are part of the reason that slow and patient anal penetration is so important. Each person's rectum and its curves are unique, and it is best to feel your way inside the rectum rather than jamming anything in there.

Beyond the rectum is the colon. The colon serves no specific sexual function, and most people never move beyond the rectum during anal penetration. However, I mention it for one important reason: the colon, rather than the rectum, is where feces are stored. They move into the rectum when you are ready to have a bowel movement. Once you go to the bathroom, there should not be any significant amount of feces left in your rectum.

Before I move on to the particulars of sexual response, a brief word about terminology. Unlike most sex educators, who are married to *penis* and *vagina* (and sometimes *clitoris*), I tend to vary the vocabulary I use to describe our genitals. In addition to these terms, which I sometimes find just too clinical sounding, I will also employ words like *pussy, clit, dick, cock,* and *ass.* I hope I don't offend you—I simply find that *pussy* rolls off my tongue more smoothly. And I don't think of any of these terms as derogatory or negative; they are simply alternatives.

The Story of O

Men have a slight to pronounced advantage over women when it comes to orgasms. By the time they are adolescents, most boys have masturbated and reached orgasm. They know how to make themselves come, and recognize the feeling when someone else helps them climax. Girls are less likely to masturbate or experience an orgasm than boys are. It may take years before they begin self-exploration and achieve their first orgasm. Unfortunately, some adult women still haven't experienced one.

If men come to me for advice because they are having difficulty making their lovers orgasm, my first question is always, "Can she have an orgasm by herself? Has she ever had an orgasm before?" It's critical to have this information before you proceed. If a woman has never experienced orgasm or has never been able to bring herself there, then it's a tremendous amount of pressure to think that someone else will be able to do it. If you have never had an orgasm before and you want to learn how to achieve one, you must dedicate yourself to self-exploration before you even attempt orgasm with a partner. I recommend reading a book, watching a video, or attending a workshop on self-loving, and, of course, practice, practice, practice!

For those of you who've already experienced the joys of the Big O, you know how it feels, but do you understand how an orgasm actually happens in the body? Sex researchers Masters and Johnson came up with a nifty little sexual response cycle divided into four phases: excitement, plateau, orgasm, and resolution.[3] If you have ever paid attention to how your body reacts during sex, then you are probably already familiar with its arousal cycle. When you first get turned on, your breathing rate and heart rate increase. Your skin may get flushed or become more sensitive in different areas. Your nipples get their own perky erections, and, for women, your breasts may swell. As blood rushes to the genital area, the clitoris and the penis become engorged and swell. A woman's inner lips also swell and may change color, and the vagina starts to lubricate and expand. Men and women's sphincter muscles react as your anus and rectum also become engorged; some people may feel the anal area relax and others may experience contractions in their sphincter muscles.

All this swelling, engorgement, erection, and expansion continue until you reach that moment just before you climax, which is called the plateau. Your blood pressure, heart rate, and breathing continue to increase. The clitoral glans swells and retreats behind the hood. Men's testicles enlarge and pull up toward the pelvis. Blood continues to rush to the genital region, and your muscle tension increases.

When you actually have an orgasm, your pelvic muscles have a series of rhythmic contractions, and the blood that has been pumping to your genitals is released. A woman's uterus also contracts. For men, orgasm and ejaculation are actually two separate occurrences, though they seem to happen simultaneously. During the resolution phase, your body eventually returns to its original, nonaroused state. The amount of time it takes varies depending on the person.

Most women (and many men) report that they don't experience an orgasm in the same way every time they have one. Women in particular may experience different sensations between one orgasm and another; they may locate the center of an orgasm in different parts of the body. An orgasm may come quickly or very slowly, last for a few seconds or several minutes. All this variety depends on what helped bring them there—clitoral stimulation, vaginal penetration, anilingus, or a combination of stimulating activities. Changes in orgasm also may be affected by a slew of different factors, including menstrual cycle, stress level, emotional state, and physical health.

Many people believe that there are actually different types of female orgasm that can be named and loosely classified. Sex researchers Beverly Whipple and John D. Perry identified three kinds: the "vulval orgasm" triggered by the clitoris, the "uterine orgasm" from vaginal intercourse, and a combination of the two.[4]

Other sexologists agree that different activities bring on different orgasms. For example, the clitoral orgasm is brought on by clitoral stimulation and is thought to be the most common type of orgasm. Other types include: the vaginal orgasm achieved through vaginal penetration; the G-spot orgasm from stimulation of the urethral sponge, which may or may not include ejaculation; the anal orgasm reached through anal penetration. Orgasm isn't an easy thing to label, however. Some women may come without being touched anywhere on their bodies, and others can have an orgasm through intense tantric breathing exercises—what do we call those orgasms? What if you combined several sensations, like clitoral stimulation and anal penetration or vaginal penetration and G-spot stimulation—how would you classify the resulting orgasms? Certain combinations of sensations may produce certain kinds of orgasms, just as that pairing of silk boxers and cologne might really put you in a certain kind of mood. Or sometimes a particular position allows for a unique angle that leads to an equally individual orgasmic experience.

Men and women have a variety of orgasmic experiences. Sometimes an orgasm can be a quick release, or sometimes it's an extended, sublime feeling that lasts for several minutes. Some orgasms are felt mainly between the legs, but others seem to resonate throughout the entire body. I am wary of naming and categorizing orgasms. Our sexual anatomical parts are so close together and all of them participate one way or another in arousal. We know that the clit doesn't just end and the G-spot begin—they are interconnected in a complex structure of tissue, nerves, blood vessels, muscles, and other structures. They all work together, so it's not necessary to give one credit over another. If they each do their part, we slide right to the edge of a cliff and over it in shuddering ecstasy. I'd say orgasms are orgasms. Call them what you like—they are undeniably some of the best feelings you will ever have.

The PC Muscle

The pelvic floor muscles play an important role in arousal and orgasm. At the bottom of the pelvic floor in both men and women is a broad, flat muscle called the pubococcygeus muscle (nicknamed the "PC muscle"). The urethra, vagina, and anus of a woman pass through this muscle, and the PC muscle surrounds a man's prostate; this muscle supports the pelvis from the pubic bone to the tailbone. Imagine that you are urinating and want to stop the flow of urine; the muscle you use to halt your pee midstream is the PC muscle. If you put your finger on your perineum while you do this, you can feel the contraction of the muscle. The PC and other pelvic muscles support the tissue of the perineum, which explains why both women and men may find this spot especially sensitive during sex. For both men and women, this muscle contracts randomly during sexual arousal and more rhythmically during orgasm.

By exercising your PC muscle, you become more in tune with the feelings in your pelvic area, thereby increasing your sensitivity and responsiveness. As with any other muscle, exercising the PC muscle tones and strengthens it, making it more flexible and more receptive to pleasurable sensations. Women and men who regularly exercise their PC muscle report many positive effects. They have increased pleasure during vaginal and anal penetration; some women can contract their PC muscle around their partner's penis, increasing sensations for her and him. Women may find they can achieve orgasm easier or faster. Men with a strong PC muscle are better able to separate orgasm from ejaculation or to delay ejaculation, both important aspects of being multiorgasmic. Both men and women have greater control over their orgasms, have better and stronger orgasms—they even have more orgasms!

Named for the scientist who studied the PC muscle and popularized the theory of exercising it, Kegel exercises can help strengthen the muscle. The most important thing to remember about Kegel exercises is to do them as regularly as possible, which shouldn't be a problem because they are pretty simple. You can do the exercises lying down, sitting, or standing—you can even do them while you're driving, riding public transportation, or sitting at your desk at work. The harder the exercises are for you to do, the less toned your PC muscles are, and the more they need a good workout. However, if you experience any pain while doing them, see a doctor.

Women and men have the ability to attain multiple orgasms, but each person is different. Women can recover more quickly from an orgasm—our bodies can get revved up all over again more easily than men's bodies can. Every woman is different when it comes to multiple orgasms. Some work hard for one great orgasm, some aren't satisfied with less than a few. You've probably known or heard of a woman so incredibly orgasmic that she could contend for an Olympic medal!

For men, the prospect of becoming multiorgasmic can be more challenging, but also very rewarding. Men who want to become multiorgasmic must first accept the fact that not every orgasm needs an erection and has to lead to ejaculation to be a bona fide come. Like women, men can have a whole range of orgasms. Once you grasp this concept, you're halfway there. Multiorgasmic men tend to climax several times without ejaculation. They learn to control, delay, and postpone ejaculation in favor of a climactic feeling.

The best way to learn to control and delay ejaculation and to climax without ejaculating is to practice various techniques while masturbating (see sidebar). It requires concentration, patience, and repetition, so why not hone your skills by yourself before you try them out with your partner? Slow, deep breathing will not only help to focus your energy and control your orgasms better, but it will decrease your heart rate. A slower heart rate can help delay orgasm. Once you feel confident, try your tricks with your partner. Women, the idea is to get him to the point of

PC Muscle Exercises

Here are a few suggestions for strengthening your PC muscles:

- Take a deep breath and while you inhale, contract the muscles and hold the contraction for a few seconds. Then exhale and relax the muscles. This combination of inhale-contract and exhale-relax is what your body does naturally. For best results, you should do about one hundred repetitions per day.

- Take a deep breath and while you inhale, tighten and release the muscles repeatedly (about ten times), then exhale and relax. Try to do these contractions quickly. Doing twenty to fifty sets a day is recommended.

- Inhale and pretend you are sucking water inside your vagina (if you've got one) and anus. Then exhale and bear down, pushing out that imaginary water. You will exercise your pelvic muscles and your stomach muscles. For best results, do ten to thirty each day.

- There is also a wonderful sex toy for women called the Kegelcisor (available at better sex toy stores), which is a vaginal barbell made of chrome-plated brass; it comes with a booklet of exercises and I highly recommend it for women interesting in developing their PC muscle.

climax. He postpones ejaculation (but still feels like he climaxed) and is ready to go again.

Because women and men experience pleasure very differently and tend to have dissimilar arousal cycles, it can be futile to chase that elusive goal that so many people inquire about in sex workshops—the simultaneous orgasm. While it sounds so

How to Keep Her Coming

- *Keep going:* Once her body shudders with orgasm number one, continue to stimulate her clitoris the way she likes it—some women can extend their orgasms if the stimulation doesn't end.

- *Switch spots:* She might like to experience an orgasm from clitoral stimulation first, then move on to vaginal penetration and G-spot stimulation. Once she has come, her G-spot will become more pronounced (easier for you to find) and more sensitive (better feeling for her).

- *Change the tune:* Her clit may feel too sensitive after an orgasm, so as you let her clit recover, try more indirect stimulation, a lighter touch, or focus on other erogenous zones until she's ready for more clitoral stimulation.

- *Let her do it:* No one knows her body better than she does. Encourage her to touch herself the second time around while you penetrate her with your fingers, your cock, or a dildo.

- *Use a toy:* You may have a stiff neck after getting her to that first orgasm, so let a vibrator take over if she's begging for more.

ideal and romantic—two lovers reaching climax at the exact same time—it can be unrealistic considering the way that our minds and bodies work. I applaud couples who want to attain simultaneous orgasm, and, of course, encourage everyone to go for what they want and have a blast trying. Usually, simultaneous orgasm involves the man delaying his orgasm. Then his partner can become more aroused and reach a similar state; in other words, he holds off so she can catch up. Timing is everything and communication is essential; couples who know each other

Making a Multiorgasmic Man

- *Press his button:* When he tells you he's close to coming, depending on the position you're in, either you or he should press on the spot on his perineum right above his anus. This ancient Taoist technique helps stop the ejaculatory reflex. If you've hit the right spot, you should feel an indentation; press about a half-inch in.

- *Tug the sac:* Place your hand at the bottom of his penis, palm down. Gently grab the scrotal sac using your thumb and forefinger and tug downward. Pulling the testicles away from the body can delay ejaculation.

- *Withdraw and squeeze:* If he's getting close, have him pull out. Place your fingers below the head of his penis and your thumb on top, then squeeze the tip of it.

- *Twenty-minute rule:* If he's learned all the techniques and is a marathon man, make sure he lets his erection go down a bit every twenty minutes so blood can circulate.

very well sexually and feel especially connected during sex often have an easier time judging where the other is at and adjusting their pace accordingly.

Striving to come at the same time and meet each other's sexual needs is a noble cause and one I support; however, I encourage people to move beyond goal-oriented sex. Sometimes, if we get too focused on results, timing, and orgasms, we lose sight of the actual experience, the intimacy we can share with a lover, the pleasure we can give one another. If you get too caught up in reaching the end, you miss out on the best parts! Relax, take your time, explore and enjoy each other's bodies without inhibition, look your partner in the eyes, and openly give and receive pleasure. That's what awesome sex is all about.

Beyond What's Between Our Legs

After reading pages and pages of information on male and female genitals, my next point may sound like a contradiction: sometimes we focus so much on our below-the-waist parts that we forget the rest of our bodies. We get so fixated on cocks and clits and pussies that we overlook plenty of other erogenous spots. Women's breasts and nipples can be extremely sensitive, and playing with them can be a big turn-on. During arousal, nipples swell, become erect, and may change color, and breasts also swell, flush, and become more receptive. People like their nipples licked, kissed, sucked, nibbled, pulled, pinched, and even bitten on occasion. It's always best to ask your partner what kind of nipple play she or he enjoys. Likewise, men's nipples are far too overlooked as a site of erotic pleasure; they too become erect and sensitive when a man is turned on, and his chest may become flushed, tingly, and more sensitive. Experiment with different sensations—a light touch, your nails, a leather glove, a piece of fur, ice cubes, and other creative textures—on chests, breasts, and nipples (see sidebar).

Although certain parts of our bodies change during sexual arousal and contribute to the arousal cycle, there are no hard and fast rules about what constitutes an erogenous zone. If it turns you on, then it's an erogenous zone. Everyone is different, and what works for one person may not do a thing for another. It's important to consider all parts of our bodies fair game when it comes to sexual excitement and stimulation. Don't discount the spark you'll cause when you brush the back of her knees. See what happens when you slide your hand up his inner thigh. If your lover has a foot fetish, then you know how good a well-rubbed (or even well-sucked) toe can feel. Trail your tongue

What to Do with Nipples

- *Lick 'em:* Trace around the outside of the nipple with your tongue. Vary the pressure of your tongue from light licks to quick flicks. Use the tip of your tongue to tease the nipple and feel it become an erect little nub in your mouth.

- *Suck 'em:* Savor a nipple like a tasty treat in your mouth. Take it between your lips and suck it gently. Vary the amount of suction, and see what elicits the best response.

- *Pull 'em:* Take a nipple between your fingers and stroke it gently. Tug it slightly, then let your fingers slip off it. Prolong your pull, watching how your partner responds. Try to delicately stretch it away from the body. Rub and roll it around in your fingers.

- *Pinch 'em:* Using your thumb and forefinger, slowly pinch the nipple, then quickly release the pressure. Increase the pressure the next time, and see how much your partner can take.

- *Nibble 'em:* Some people like a little teeth in the mix. Best to start with a slight nibble at first and work your way up. Biting can be delicious or downright painful, depending on the person, so make sure you ask before you clamp down with those pearly whites.

- *Clamp 'em:* Speaking of clamps, if your partner likes pinching and biting, you may want to kick it up a notch. You can use clothespins or nipple clamps, which you can buy at sex-toy stores (see chapter 9 for more on nipple clamps).

along the back of her neck, nibble on his earlobes, rub the tip of your finger on her lips. The idea is to explore your partner's body with plenty of eagerness and willingness (and hey, explore your own while you masturbate!).

And let us not forget one of the most important erogenous zones we have: the brain. Nestled inside the skull, the brain controls sexual functioning. What happens in our minds is just as important as what's rubbing up against our genitals, and there are many factors that affect a person's experience of sex. Although I resist many generalizations based on gender, the emotional aspects of sex affect women more than men. Of course, this isn't a universal truth, and some of the following observations can hold true for both Tarzan and Jane. A woman's sexual self-image and how she feels about her body both contribute to how she relates to her partner. The emotional connection between partners as well as the nature, status, and security of the relationship also play an important role in how a woman feels about sex. Psychological elements, including her expectations, anxieties, and fantasies, weave their way between the bedsheets as well. The power dynamics between partners, the context of the sexual encounter, and even past sexual experiences are also significant to women's sexual enjoyment. A woman's overall mental-health and stress level can deeply affect her sexual pleasure.

Because our minds and hearts are so critical to our pleasure, even the most practiced and finessed physical techniques may not do the trick. That's why, above all else, it is so important to communicate with your partner, discover each other's sexual desires and fantasies, and listen to each other with love and respect.

My wife is five months pregnant, and this is our first child. Her desire for sex fluctuates, but I want to know if it is safe to have sex all the way through nine months. Is there anything we shouldn't do that might hurt the baby?

Throughout her pregnancy, penetrating her (both vaginally and anally) with your fingers is safe; penetration with your penis is safe in low-risk pregnancies. After she becomes pregnant, she may feel that her orgasms change—don't worry, that's common. One of the challenges of sex during pregnancy is finding comfortable positions; experiment and see what works for both of you. Avoid deep thrusting and really hard slamming of any kind. Using water-based lubricants is fine, but a word of caution about anal play: be extra careful in preventing bacteria from the ass transferring to the vagina. Keep fingers and toys super clean, or she may get an infection, which is often harder to treat during pregnancy. Oral sex is fine, but never blow air in the vagina; this can cause a serious condition and threaten the mother's life. Avoid anything that might bruise the cervix (including deep thrusting). If she feels any discomfort during any sexual activity, stop at once.

TELL ME WHAT YOU WANT

Erotic Desire,
Sexual Communication,
and Safer Sex

Discovering Your Desire

Knowing what you want—and what you don't—is the first step to getting it. Discovering your desires is a key ingredient to having a satisfying sexual relationship, but that task is sometimes easier said than done. There are many barriers that can prevent us from listening to our own hearts. Our parents may (or may not) sit down with us to have that "birds and bees" talk, but rarely does anyone teach us how to determine what we want to do or how to do it. From *Cosmopolitan,* romance novels, and soap operas to *Esquire,* mainstream movies, and adult videos, the media saturates us with images and ideas of what we *should* want, things like romance, silk sheets, or soft lighting. Popular images convey what we *could* have: a *Baywatch* lifeguard, a supermodel, or a movie star. Rarely does that same media encourage us to discover our own distinct desires.

Desire is as unique as the individual, and it cannot be neatly packaged in a half-hour sitcom or a one-page quiz in a women's magazine. So how do you go about figuring out what makes you tick sexually, what gets the motor revved up and the engine humming? Sexual desire is a complex combination of physical, emotional, psychological, and even spiritual elements. The trick is to figure out what all the different elements are for *you.*

People who are very conscious of their emotions probably have an idea of how feelings factor into their sex lives. For others, you might have to dig a little to become aware of how your emotional needs play a significant role in determining your sexual needs. A desire to please, to be perfect, to feel safe, to be wanted, to be in control—people often meet these emotional needs and a whole slew of others through sex. Feeling cared for and loved, making a connection, and trusting your partner can be critical to sexual desire. Often if you are fighting with your partner or some issue has gone undiscussed or unresolved, your sexual desire diminishes. Metaphorically speaking, we often want to make love in a clean bed. Think back to some of the most satisfying sex you've ever had, and remember the emotional relationship. Beyond the physical sensations, how did you *feel* when you had sex? It will give you great insight into your emotional desire.

Psychologically, we also have different needs when it comes to sex. Some people want to feel like they are being "taken" by their partners, surrendering, or losing control. Others like to initiate sex, be the one in charge calling the shots. And still others switch back and forth between these roles depending on their mood. Again, it often helps to reflect on past sexual relationships—what dynamics between you and your lover fueled the passion? When you watch a romantic scene in a film or read an erotic story, think about whom you most identify with—is it the aggressor, the shy lover, the dominatrix, the sexually voracious partner, the virgin, or the teacher? Characters you see yourself in will give you clues to your psychological roles in sex. Also consider which characters attract you. If you are attracted to the handsome charmer, you probably enjoy being charmed. If the mysterious stranger turns you on, you might like a little danger with your sex. If someone inexperienced appeals to you, then I bet you've got some initiation fantasies. Once you explore how you experience sex on an emotional and psychological level, you can better understand how these intangible elements affect your sex life.

In order to find out what turns you on, the first and best place to start is with yourself. Masturbation is one of the best gifts you can give yourself—it can be not only satisfying and enjoyable, but a learning experience as well. A lot of times, especially when we are in relationships, we get lazy about self-love. You should really make a date once a week (or more) to get back in *touch* with yourself. One of the best ways to become a better lover is to know your own body and sexuality in the deepest and fullest way possible. The more knowledge you have, the easier it will be to clue your partner in to your unique erotic self. The more aware you are of your own body and its capacity for pleasure, the more you will be able to receive, enjoy, and revel in that pleasure when it comes from another person. Masturbation is a super way to explore, rediscover, and study the erogenous zones, sweet spots, and sensitive areas of your body. Pay attention to how you make yourself come. What sends you into overdrive—a particular kind of touch or pressure, a favorite sex toy, a surefire position? Study your own techniques, so you can teach them to your lover later. The physical tricks can be just as important as the emotional ones when it comes right down to it. If you can please yourself, you can usually get someone else to please you (with a little practice, of course!).

You also may want to make a list of what your favorite sexual activities with your partner are currently, and be as specific as you can. For example: vaginal penetration in doggie-style position with him reaching around to rub your clit; deep kissing for a long time leading up to sex; an extended blow job where she teases you a lot and licks your balls; cunnilingus with you straddling his face and him playing with your ass.

While you are masturbating, you can also discover some of

Clues from Past Sex

Think, meditate, or write in a journal about your past sexual experiences; they may give you a window into your desires. Use these superlatives as a guideline for remembering instances, then delve into them and explore what about them made them great.

- Your Most Romantic Sexual Experience

- Your Most Passionate Sexual Experience

- Your Most Uninhibited Sexual Experience

- Your Most Fun Sexual Experience

- Your Most Intense Sexual Experience

- Your Most Kinky Sexual Experience

your nonphysical turn-ons if you start to become aware of what comes to mind. Are there specific images that get the juices flowing? Do you fantasize about people you know, strangers, or celebrities? Are there particular scenarios that turn you on and drive you wild? Can some of your fantasies be acted out in the real world? Remember that desires are your own, they may not be racy or on the edge, they may not be sweet or politically correct, but they are yours. Cut yourself some slack and let them be what they are.

There are many different components to desire. You may have favorite physical activities like oral sex, anal sex, or mutual masturbation. You may want to try a new position, a new lube, a new technique, or a new sex toy. Perhaps your taste is for something more out of the ordinary, like bondage or spanking. Maybe your fantasies involve role-playing particular scenarios.

Whatever it is, doing something just because you think you should is never a good idea. Do it because you want to do it and the desire is authentic, not because it's something you think everyone else is doing or your partner is pressuring you to do. Tap into your own desires, claim them, unleash them! In an ideal world, your partner is your mirror opposite, and your desires meld with each other perfectly. But, more likely, your desires will come together in not-so-perfect-but-we-can-make-it-work harmony. The best way to know if your desires are compatible is to talk about them.

Talking Before Sex

Communication before, during, and after sex is crucial to having a satisfying relationship. While it may be difficult, talking to your partner, sharing your desires, fantasies, and even your fears, will greatly enhance your intimacy as a couple. As with everything else, start out slowly and gently. Ask yourself and your partner: What do you want out of our sexual relationship? What do you expect from sex? Having an open, honest discussion can help illuminate what each person desires, so both people are less likely to make incorrect assumptions about the other person's expectations. Learning to talk about sex openly and honestly takes practice. One way to start the process of talking is to keep a journal, where you can write about sex. The idea behind keeping a journal is that if you can write about your feelings about sex, eventually you'll have the nerve to say them out loud, too. You could skip the writing part altogether, of course, and just start talking. The more you do it, the easier it will get. Remember that your lover knows you well, but no one is a mind reader. You have to take responsibility for finding out what your desires are, sharing them with your partner, and working together to fulfill them.

Talking about sex in a nonsexual context is often easier than doing it in bed just before a little midnight romp. Take the pres-

Starting a Conversation About Sex

Finish these sentences to yourself, in a journal or face-to-face with your partner:

- What I love most about having sex with you is . . .

- You turn me on when you . . .

- One of the best times we had sex was . . . because . . .

- When I want to have sex and you don't, I feel . . .

- To feel like I am in the mood for sex, I need . . .

- When we have oral sex (or fill in the blank with whatever you want), I feel . . .

- If I could ask you to do one thing to me the next time we have sex, I would like you to . . .

sure off yourself and your partner by bringing up difficult issues or new topics in a totally neutral environment. Make sure you are in a place where you can talk freely. Sex talks are nearly impossible to have in your mother-in-law's living room, with the kids running in and out of the room, or at the grocery store (unless you've checked and your aisle is clear!). People always ask me: "How do I approach a sexual subject with my part- ner—like something new I'd like to try—when I don't know how he or she will react?" Again, choose a neutral time and place where your partner won't feel pressured or threatened by this new revelation. Sometimes, people feel more comfortable first approaching the subject in an indirect or "hypothetical" way. For example: "I just read about a book on anal sex for women—what do you think about that?" or "A friend of Susan's says she and her boyfriend have been experimenting with bondage and blindfolds . . ." Of course, there is also always the direct approach, which I favor and applaud, but I realize that not everyone is there yet.

Maybe you have a concern about sex, a worry about what your partner thinks about your desires, or an anxiety about a particular activity. If you feel pressure or guilt, these and other negative emotions can not only mess with your head, they can also manifest themselves on a physical level and interfere with your enjoyment of sex. An honest discussion before sex gives both of you a chance to air concerns, alleviate fears, and reassure each other. The more secure and positive you feel, the better your sex life will be.

Communication During Sex

It's tragic that too many people are still having sex in the dark without saying one word to each other. How can you possibly know what the other person wants if he or she isn't giving you a clue? One and only one person holds the key to your pleasure: you, and you need to speak up! You can approach verbal communication with your partner during sex in several ways.

"Straight" Talk During Sex

Talking during sex can enrich the experience in many different ways. First and foremost, both partners can feel they've been given some direction and aren't simply flying blind. A lover armed with information can proceed with a sense of security that he likes that, she asked for this, that feels good. Information can be a beautiful thing. Second, you can give and receive feedback about what you're doing. For instance, say your partner asks you to stimulate her clitoris. Well, you can do it a bunch of different ways. With feedback, she can be more specific and you can feel better instructed: *When I say more pressure, I mean like this.*

I like the vibrator, but I want it right here. Move your tongue up and down instead of side to side. You can also get some feedback on what you're *not* doing. Like: *Baby, play with my nipples. I want your fingers inside me when you're going down on me. Put your hand here when you are sucking my dick.* A back-and-forth dialogue during the deed can also provide much-needed validation that you are giving your partner pleasure, reassurance that all lovers crave and appreciate. Encouragement makes us feel good, pumps us up, and gives us confidence to go the extra mile and make our lovers scream like banshees!

Lovers new to one another can't be expected to know or even guess correctly what someone likes or doesn't like sexually. That's why we need to tell them. The object of the game here is to communicate as clearly as possible and without judgment or condescension. For the most part, people like instruction and guidance. I've found that if you tell someone what to do—and you aren't patronizing or ego-trampling about it—they'll do it. People want directions. The funny thing is that almost everything in our lives comes with instructions—the VCR, the computer, our jobs—but people don't come with manuals when they get into our beds. And if they did, remember each manual would be completely unique to that person. Be as specific as possible in your cues: *a little to the left, softer, deeper, slower.* This can also be an opportunity to *show* your partner exactly what you mean by demonstrating it on yourself or guiding some part of their body over some part of yours.

If your partner is shy about speaking up during sex, you may need to coax or prompt a little. Ask simple, straightforward questions during the deed. *Do you want it faster? Is this position working for you? Do you want more direct pressure on your clit?* Or the ever-popular *how does that feel?*

Dirty Talk

Speaking of *how does that feel?*, that simple question and its answer can also be the beginning of a less informational and more down-and-dirty dialogue during sex. It's all in the way you say it. Erotic talk doesn't have to be "dirty" per se—it can be sweet, sensual, and romantic, or it can be bold, nasty, and raunchy. Whichever way you say it, dirty talk can heighten a sexual experience and really drive both of you over the edge.

Most people are interested in dabbling in some hot conversation, but don't know how to start the fire. The easiest way to begin is to describe what's going on. This may seem like simply stating the obvious, but you'd be surprised at how much of a turn-on the most basic sex talk can be. Frank sexual descriptions are not usually part of everyday discussion, so "saying it loud" can be titillating, provocative, and even a little naughty. Especially if you put it in such a way that it sounds breathy, passionate, or downright nasty. For example: "You're so wet. I've got my dick inside that wet hole of yours and it feels great." Talk about what you are doing, what you are going to do, what you want to do. Like: "Honey, put my cock in your mouth. I really want to feel your lips around me." Tease, tempt, torment a little: "I'm gonna lick your pussy and get you all worked up and leave you here all turned on with no release. Do you want it? Do you?" Ask for what you want, beg for what you need: "I'm gonna go crazy if you don't put your fingers in my ass right now. Please . . ." Some people like to actually spin out a whole story or scenario to complement what's going on physically. Tell an erotic story, share a fantasy about what you were thinking about doing to your partner all day while at work, describe something you saw in an erotic video, and how you'd like to try it with your partner.

Sexy talk takes practice, and it's probably best for beginners to start simple. Fear, embarrassment, or shyness can prevent you from opening your mouth in the first place. Reassure yourself and your partner that it's safe to talk, and no one will be criti-

Dirty Talk Tips

- *Describe:* The simple act of narrating your sexual encounter can be sexier than you may think.

- *Instruct:* Some people not only appreciate being told what to do, it turns them on. Get in touch with your inner dominatrix, and dole out an order or two.

- *Be naughty:* Think of the wildest stuff you've always wanted to say and go for it. Channel your inner bad boy or bad girl.

- *Beg:* Desperation is normally not very sexy, but when you are desperate for your partner to do something, a little begging can go a long way.

- *Be outrageous:* Let your inhibitions go, and let the sexual banter flow! Be bold and bawdy, let your mind wander and your mouth follow.

- *Tease:* This can be an incredibly effective verbal turn-on. Tell her what you're going to do to her, then make her wait. Couple your words with a few suggestive touches, and you'll whip her into a frenzy.

- *Tell a Story:* Now is your chance to create that erotic story you've been dreaming about or put you and your lover in a porn-movie encounter.

cized or chastised for what comes out of their mouth. You also need to test the waters with your partner about just how raunchy you can get (and this might be a good thing to bring up before you open your mouth). For some, words like "cunt" and "slut" are a total turn-on, while for others, those same words seem vulgar and defeat the purpose of arousal altogether. Don't force dirty talk, let it flow out of your mouth as naturally as juice flows from a pussy. Say what's on your mind; honesty can be the hottest thing around. Once you get into it, let your inhibitions go. You'll be talking up a storm in no time!

Of course, straight talk and dirty talk are not mutually exclusive. You can create your own dialogue which both instructs and arouses, or you can move back and forth between giving straight information and whispering nasty little thoughts. You can stick to one, then the next time try the other. Change your tone of voice ever so slightly, and go from nice to naughty in ten seconds flat. Whatever the case, give yourself permission and plenty of space to open your mouth and speak your mind. You might just be surprised what comes out.

Talking After Sex

As you recover from orgasm, lying together sweaty and sticky, you may or may not feel much like talking. But there is a reason that secret agents are debriefed after an important mission. Having as much information as possible puts them in a powerful position. When your mission is great sex, you too need a debriefing session. Perhaps the afterglow of lovemaking is not the best time for one. Wait a little while and bring it up when you both have the time and energy to talk about it. I don't mean for you to overanalyze each of your sex sessions or process them blow-by-blow every single time. But shortly after fucking is a good time to talk about fucking. It's a great way to be specific while the details of the encounter are still fresh in both your minds.

You can talk about what turned you on, what felt really good, what you could do without next time, what you'd like more of, what could go on a little longer (hint, hint), something that surprised you, something you thought of during sex, something you'd like to try next time. You can use these examples in the form of questions in order to gather information about your partner's feelings about your sex life. For example: *What turned you on? What would you like more of?* And so on. Sometimes people who are shy about talking explicitly about sex respond better to specific questions, rather than the old, "So how was it for you?" To which the tight-lipped will often respond, "Fine," which doesn't give you much to go on. Probe as gently as possible for more information by asking specific questions: "Did you like it when I sucked your cock like that?" "When I am licking your pussy, do you want me to put a few fingers inside you?"

In general, be generous and caring when you communicate with your partner. When you want to bring up something you don't like, remember: compliments always feel good—criticism does not. If you want to tell her about something you didn't like, why not start that conversation with something you did like? Make sure to talk about what wasn't pleasurable as well as what was pleasurable. The more you talk about it, the easier it will get. Trust me.

Talking About Safer Sex

There is another part of sexual communication that is difficult, but necessary: negotiating safer sex practices. Discussing your sexual history, your health, and your feelings about safer sex may not be fun and titillating, but it's very important. It will also put your mind at ease.

Even if you are in a monogamous relationship, the American Medical Women's Association recommends that you and your partner should be tested for HIV six months after you or your partner has had sexual contact with a different partner.[5] During that six-month period, you should practice safer sex. Get tested for STDs like herpes, gonorrhea, chlamydia, and syphilis. Consider being tested for hepatitis if you are at risk. If you and your partner are monogamous and disease-free, and your six months have passed, you may choose not to use any barriers at all during sex, although you may still use condoms as birth control or latex gloves for easier clean up.

If you have multiple partners, then you should practice safer sex with all of them to prevent sexually transmitted diseases and HIV/AIDS. Some couples agree to regularly swap bodily fluids with each other (sometimes called "fluid bonding"), but are nonmonogamous because they also have additional sex partners. These fluid-bonded partners still practice safer sex with all other sexual partners.

The following sexual activities are considered relatively low risk: deep French kissing, frottage or rubbing, fellatio with a condom, vaginal or anal penetration with fingers using a glove, manual stimulation of clitoris, vagina, or penis, cunnilingus with a barrier. Unprotected cunnilingus (not during menstruation), vaginal or anal penetration with ungloved fingers, and unprotected fellatio are all considered risky, and the risk is higher with ejaculation in the mouth. High-risk activities include: unprotected cunnilingus during menstruation, unprotected oral/anal contact; unprotected vaginal intercourse; unprotected anal intercourse; and sharing sex toys without a condom.

Protecting yourself during cunnilingus and anilingus means putting a barrier between your mouth and your partner's genitals. Originally designed for use by dentists, as the name indicates, dental dams are squares of latex which safer-sex practitioners have co-opted for use as oral sex barriers. Because they were not developed with sex in mind, dental dams can be too small and too thick to make them ideal. Glyde Dams are a larger, thinner version designed specifically for oral sex which do the job much better than traditional dental dams. They are available at better sex-toy stores. (See the Resource Guide for more information.)

To make your own latex dam, you can cut a nonlubricated condom up one side; these tend to be thinner, like the Glydes, which allows both partners more feeling and greater sensitivity.

You can also transform a latex glove into a dam: cut the wrist, the pinky side, and the fingers off, leaving the thumb intact. Open it up, stick your tongue in the thumb slot, and voilà—it's like a condom for your tongue! This is my favorite kind of a dam because it affords both giver and receiver the highest sensitivity. For obvious reasons, it's best to use a glove that isn't powdered or to rinse the powder off before you put your mouth near it. Try putting a dab of lube on the inside and outside of the thumb for even more sensitivity.

Store-bought plastic wrap (like Saran Wrap) is not just for leftovers—it also makes a good barrier for cunnilingus and anilingus. Plastic wrap is less expensive and easier to find than latex dams, which makes it more convenient. Another advantage: trying wrapping your sweetie's privates in plastic—think of it as a homemade thong. Then you can go to town without having to hold the dam in place. Safe, hands-free muff diving and ass licking at last!

To practice safer fellatio, men should wear a condom. Non-lubricated or flavored condoms are best, since the taste of a lubricated condom (many of them contain Nonoxynol-9) is not only awful, it can numb your mouth. A desensitized mouth can obviously not do its best work. Try using some lube (either flavored or with a taste you can tolerate) on the inside and outside of the condom; it will increase his feeling as well as her ability to give an expert blow job.

Putting a latex glove on your hand for finger fucking protects both you and your partner, especially if you have any cuts, scratches, or even torn cuticles which may provide an opportunity for disease transmission. Gloves come in several different sizes, and you should make sure that they fit well. A glove that's too small will cut off your circulation, and one that is too big will feel baggy and uncomfortable inside the receptive partner. You can also wear gloves for other purposes: if your nails are long, sharp, or ragged, if you are squeamish about the cleanliness of anal penetration, or if you want to smooth out your fingers before they go inside your lover. If you find that wearing latex gloves irritates your skin, you may be sensitive to the powder that coats the inside, which is common; find an unpowdered glove instead. If you are allergic to latex, look for gloves made of vinyl or other alternative materials.

As part of safer sex, you should use a condom every time you have either vaginal or anal penetration. In fact, because of the delicacy of anal and rectal tissue, bodily fluids infccted with HIV and other viruses are transmitted and absorbed more easily and quickly into the bloodstream through the mucous membrane of the rectum. Thus, unprotected anal intercourse can be more risky for both partners than unprotected vaginal intercourse.

Speaking of anal penetration, you should never, ever put anything in the vagina that has been in the anus without thoroughly washing and disinfecting it first. Transferring rectal bacteria into the vagina can lead to yeast infections, urinary tract infections, and other ailments which will put a halt to your sex life. Just don't go there. If you're likely to want to use the same hand or tool in both the vagina and the anus, or your anus and then your partner's, that's a lot of running to the bathroom to wash up each time you want to switch gears. Using a new glove and/or condom each time you switch orifices or activities means less time cleaning and more time fucking.

All About Condoms

The condom market has just exploded in the past decade. You can now find condoms with a variety of features, including: regular and extra-sensitive; lubed and nonlubed; snugger fitting and extra-large; ribbed, studded, and textured in other ways; brightly colored, black, and crystal clear; thin, thinner, and extra-thin. Your friends, lovers, and sex-toy store clerks may have some helpful recommendations, but also realize that the choice of condom is a very individual one. Many brands are sold singly

A Guide to Condoms

Bigger: Beyond Seven, Maxx, Trojan Magnum

Clear: Atlas, Durex, Trojan Supra

Colors: Midnight Desire, Lifestyles Colors, Lifestyles Tuxedo, Ria

Extra-Strong: Contempo Power Play, Lifestyles Xtra Strength

Extra-Thin: Kimono Microthin, Paradise Super Sensitive, Sagami Vis à Vis, Skinless Skin, Trojan Supra, Trojan Ultra Pleasure, Trojan Ultra Thin

Female Condom: Reality

Flavored: Lifestyles Kiss of Mint, Trustex

High Sensitivity for Him: InSpiral, Kimono Sensations, Lifestyles Ultra Sensitive, Lifestyles Xtra Pleasure, Pleasure Plus, Trojan Pleasure Mesh, Trojan Supra, Trojan Ultra Pleasure, Trojan Very Sensitive

Nonlatex: Avanti, Trojan Naturalamb, Trojan Supra

Nonlubricated: Lifestyles Non-Lubricated, Ria, Trojan Non-Lubed

Snugger: Exotica, Prime

Textured for Her: Lifestyles Ribbed, Lifestyles Rough Rider, Sagami Type E, Trojan Pleasure Mesh, Trojan Ribbed

Thin: Crown, Kimono

at sex-toy stores, so you can buy one of each and find your favorite.

If you use a condom with a receptacle tip, gently press the air out of the closed end before putting it on. Air bubbles can lead to condoms rupturing. If you use a condom with a plain end, leave about an inch of air-free space at the tip of the condom; semen needs somewhere to go and ejaculation without that space can cause a condom to break. Putting a small amount of lube on the inside tip of the condom will reduce air bubbles and increase sensitivity. Another good tip: hold onto the base of the condom when necessary, and especially during withdrawal, so it doesn't slip off. You can also use condoms on vibrators, dildos, and other sex toys to keep them clean in order to share them safely with a partner.

Marketed primarily for vaginal intercourse, the Reality Female Condom is a tube of polyurethane closed at one end and open at the other, like a larger version of the regular condom. Although some women find them cumbersome, others say it gives them a sense of control and responsibility in the practice of safer sex. The female condom can also be used for anal intercourse.

Before insertion, lubricate the outside of the condom, and make sure that the lubrication is evenly spread by rubbing the outside of the pouch together. To insert it, squeeze the sheath, and, starting with the inner ring, slip it into the vagina or the anus. Once it is inside, push it the rest of the way with your finger. About an inch of the condom should hang outside the opening, so the outer ring doesn't slip inside during the action.

During penetration, the Female Condom may move around, either side to side or up and down; this is normal, though the outer ring should never slip into the vagina or the anus. If it does, stop and adjust it. To take the condom out, squeeze and twist the outer ring (to keep fluid inside the pouch) and pull it out slowly and gently.

If you are sensitive or allergic to latex, you can still practice safer sex. Look for nonlatex condoms like Durex by Avanti. You can also use natural or lambskin condoms, but know they have a higher breakage rate than those made of latex. Use nitrile, vinyl, and polyurethane gloves instead of latex ones. They are more difficult to find, but try a medical supply store. For oral sex barriers, use plastic wrap like Saran Wrap.

Whenever you use a latex or nonlatex barrier, you should always use a lubricant with it. Lube makes safer sex smoother and more comfortable for both partners, especially for the person on the receiving end of penetration; of course, the

Making Safer Sex Hot

- *Use some lube:* The slippery stuff makes all kinds of sexual activities with latex, including penetration, smoother and more comfortable. Add lube on both sides of a latex condom or dam for better safe oral sex.

- *Add some flavor:* Lapping up the taste of latex isn't exactly enticing. Try condoms, dams, and lube in a variety of flavors, and make your mouth happy.

- *A touch of color:* Plain latex can feel too sterile and medical to make using it sexy. Luckily, condoms, dams, and gloves come in a variety of colors, which can brighten up your day, and won't remind you of a trip to the emergency room.

- *Learn to put a condom on with your mouth:* Practice on a banana or a dildo privately, then impress him with your newfound skill!

- *Make it part of seduction:* Rather than fumbling and groaning when it's time to whip out and slip on your latex friends, try making the act of slipping on a condom or a glove a hint of things to come. Think of it as a reverse strip tease.

smoother things tend to go, the more pleasurable the experience for everyone.

Nonoxynol-9, which is found in some lubricants and many lubricated condoms (read ingredients carefully), is a chemical proven to kill HIV (the virus that causes AIDS) and some STD viruses. Although it was once widely accepted that Nonoxynol-9 should be used during vaginal and anal intercourse, many women are sensitive or allergic to this harsh chemical, and develop irritation, burning, itching, even infections from it. In addition, many sex educators believe that because it's likely to irritate or traumatize the vaginal or rectal tissue, Nonoxynol-9 may actually make transmission of HIV faster and easier during intercourse, providing the virus with an accessible route to the bloodstream.[6] Recently, an international study found that women who used Nonoxynol-9 frequently were more prone to genital ulcers, and more likely to be infected with HIV as a result.[7] Genital ulcers or not, I think Nonoxynol-9 is too irritating and women should stick to a lubricant without it.

Practicing safer sex for some, all, or no sexual activities is an individual choice. We are all adults who need to assess our specific situations, think about the risks associated with what we do, and make an informed decision about protecting ourselves. If you want more information on STDs, HIV, and safer sex, ask your doctor or health care provider.

I am in my early thirties, and my sex drive seems to have decreased quite drastically—I am practically never in the mood for sex anymore, and my husband complains that I no longer initiate it. What's wrong with me?

With the discovery of Viagra, many men have found relief from erectile dysfunction and other sexual problems. Certainly there are men with other conditions that cannot be fixed with a little blue pill, but, in general, medicine knows a lot more about male sexual dysfunction. Women's sexual desire and sex drive are so unique and complex that it makes sense that our sexual dysfunction is equally complicated.

For women, a lack of sexual desire is a serious problem that may have a variety of causes, some of which we still haven't completely figured out. There may be some underlying psychological factors contributing to your lack of libido, including linger-ing shame and guilt about sex and self-esteem or body issues. Or you may have past sexual experiences, especially painful or neg-ative ones, which can have a tremendous impact on your cur-rent sexual relationship, including a history of abuse.

If your current relationship feels unstable to you, it also may be affecting your libido. If you have unresolved problems or unspoken anger, it can affect your sexual relationship as well. Plus, there are plenty of physical conditions and symptoms which serve to dampen our sex drive, including: anxiety, depres-sion, chronic fatigue, disability, pregnancy, perimenopause, menopause, stress, and many others. You may be taking med-ication—especially antidepressants—which have the unfortu-nate side effect of decreasing libido. And, of course, there may be a combination of emotional, psychological, and physical issues which come together to kill your sex drive.

Depending on what the particulars of your situation are, you have a variety of treatment options. You can consult your doctor about possibly changing any medication that may be causing the problem. Recently, some experts have recommended low doses of testosterone for women with sexual dysfunction; there are side effects, so do plenty of research before you choose this route. Because Viagra has had only mixed results for women, research-ers have been trying to come up with other more effective solu-tions, including several creams that increase blood flow and genital engorgement, which may result in increased arousal.

Some women seek out sex therapy to address the problem and learn some behavioral changes that can help. There are also several holistic and homeopathic approaches, including chiro-practic care, acupuncture, and herbs like yohimbine, saw pal-metto, and ginseng. Even though these herbs are natural, you still should see a health-care professional—do not try to self-medicate, even with herbal remedies, and always tell whoever is caring for you what medications you're taking.

Talk to your doctor to find out all your different options, and do some research yourself. I recommend three useful books: *Beyond Viagra: A Commonsense Guide to Building a Healthy Sexual Relationship for Both Men and Women,* by Dr. Gerald A. Melchiode, *I'm Not in the Mood: What Every Woman Should Know About Improving Her Libido,* by Dr. Judith Reichman, and *For Women Only: A Revolutionary Guide to Overcoming Sexual Dysfunction and Reclaiming Your Sex Life,* by Jennifer Berman, M.D., and Laura Berman, Ph.D.

MAKING THE BASICS
EVEN BETTER

Hand Jobs and Oral Sex

In the title of this chapter, I refer to hand jobs and oral sex as the basics because these activities—manual and oral stimulation of the penis, clitoris, vagina, and anus—are not as out of the ordinary as some of the others I cover later in the book. And to most people, they certainly aren't new. But just because they are basic, that doesn't mean that hand jobs and mouth jobs are simple. They require as much skill, enthusiasm, and creativity as any other form of sex, and you can teach an old dog new tricks when it comes to hands and mouths.

Also, being basic does not make manual and oral sex less enjoyable or satisfying. I want to challenge you to see these practices in a different way; they are not just hoops you've got to jump through to get to the prize (i.e., intercourse). Too often, they are relegated to being appetizers, so we don't spend enough time on them, because we want to get to the main course. Cunnilingus and fellatio can be stimulating and satisfying activities in and of themselves. What if you were to spend one evening where you could do absolutely anything you wanted to each other except have intercourse? What would you do? How would you explore each other's bodies differently? What kinds of thing would you like to do to your lover? What would you want done to you? What would bring you to orgasm?

Hand Jobs for Her

Men sometimes overlook the power they hold in their hands to give pleasure to their partners. Since both men and women masturbate using their own digits, it makes sense that women would enjoy manual stimulation with a partner. A well-delivered hand job can help you gauge her arousal level, warm her up for intercourse, or bring her to orgasm all by itself.

Don't go to her pussy right off the bat; kiss her, touch her, and wait until she's riled up a little. If she starts thrusting herself against your leg or you feel her panties get damp, you'll know she's ready for you to travel south of the border. First and foremost, men should ask their partners what kind of manual stimulation they like. It's safe to assume she wants you to focus on the clitoral glans, but every woman is different, and it never hurts to ask. Be slow and gentle at first, and keep in mind that before a woman is completely aroused, her clitoris can be too sensitive for vigorous rubbing. So begin by indirectly stimulating her clit: rub the side of her hood, rather than directly on it.

As she gets more revved up and her clitoris swells, you can increase the rubbing, and you can move directly to her clit. Experiment with different levels of pressure and motion; some women prefer an up-and-down motion, others like side-to-side rubbing or a circular movement. There is nothing worse than a dry rub, so I recommend using plenty of lube for the optimum hand job (read all about lube in chapter 4). If she feels comfortable doing it, you may ask her to show you how she likes it—then she can place her hand over yours and guide you. Remember: if anyone knows how to do her best, it's her.

Even as you're paying attention to her clit, don't ignore the rest of her pussy—rub her labia, her vaginal opening, her perineum. If she wants penetration, slowly slip a well-lubricated finger inside her, and curve it toward her navel to stimulate her G-spot (check out plenty more G-spot tips in chapter 5). Move in and out with consistent, deliberate strokes. Ask her if she wants more fingers, or if she likes it faster, harder, or deeper. Use your thumb or the palm of your hand to continue to stimulate her clit while your fingers are inside her. Make sure your nails are clean and well-trimmed; you wouldn't believe how many women have complained to me about that! Never jam your fingers inside her pussy or wander aimlessly like you are picking fruit or something. The key here is smooth, rhythmic motion. And always know that the hand job doesn't have to stop: it can and hopefully will continue during intercourse.

Hand Jobs for Him

Too many women feel frustrated, intimidated, or unmotivated to give a guy a good hand job. Women say they don't know how to do it, and, unfortunately, no one ever showed them the way. Some women believe that their partner can give himself the best hand job of all, so how could hers ever compete? Or women just dismiss the hand job as something a high school girl might do, an inferior, adolescent act they've moved beyond. Remember that a well-executed hand job can be titillating, pleasurable, and fun for both partners.

The first thing women need to know about is something that will drastically improve their technique: lubricant. That's right, just a few squirts of lube on your hand, and you'll be on your way to working his cock well. Lube helps you make one smooth motion which obviously feels much better than a dry run up and down the pole. The trick is to achieve slickness and friction at once, and when you've greased the runway, it's much easier to accomplish. As with anything else, when women ask their male

Hand Jobs Tricks for Him and Her

- *Jiffy Lube:* Add some lube to the equation.

- *Watch and Learn:* Have your partner show you what he or she likes.

- *Hot Spots:* For him, the head of the penis; for her, the clitoris.

- *Full Body:* Don't ignore nipples, lips, inner thighs, butt, and the rest of the body.

- *Open Mouth:* Hey, it's one advantage over oral sex—your mouth isn't full! So use it to talk dirty or tell your lover what you like.

partners what they like—or watch as he demonstrates his techniques—they feel more confident and excited about doing it because they are closer to doing it well. Women should experiment with different levels of pressure to see what feels best to him, minding long nails, so they don't scratch him. Pay close attention to the most sensitive part of his cock, the head. And don't forget about the rest of his body—play with his testicles, tweak his nipples, hey, you could even squeeze his ass.

Pussy Licking

First and foremost, oral sex should be fun for both the giver and the recipient. Guys, women can usually tell if you're not into going down on them, so don't do them any favors if you aren't going to give your all. Effort and enthusiasm are always appreciated. Throw yourself into it and she'll love you for it. But, while you may get an A for enthusiasm, skill and technique count toward your average, so study up. Before your mouth is full, you may want to ask her for some pointers. You can't tell how a woman wants her pussy licked just by looking at her, and chances are, the tricks that worked on your last lover will only get you so far with this one.

Like the hand job, don't rush to rug munching—your tongue techniques will feel so much better for her when she's turned on. Start by licking all around her pussy, waking her up and beginning the arousal process. When you've warmed her up, and she's juicy and swollen, concentrate on her clitoris. Alternate between different kinds of strokes: up and down, side to side, circular, and figure eights. Try making big, thick licks from the top of her clitoral hood all the way down to her perineum, and back up again. Be creative with your tongue, lips, and mouth. Some women like you to suck on their clitoris; do it gently at first to see if she's one of them. Explore different strokes and amounts of pressure.

If you want to add penetration to the mix, lube up your finger and slip inside her while your tongue works her clit. Remember to aim for that G-spot; you can even try to gently "scratch your tongue" from inside her. If your partner likes more than average pressure on her clit, try using your nose to give her the fix she craves. All the variety will help keep her entertained and give you some idea about which of your tricks work best, but at some point you're going to have to commit to one thing and stick to it to make her come—once again, rhythm and consistency will get her to ecstasy. Listen to her body. If she shoves her pussy into you, then chances are she wants more or harder or both. If she rocks her hips away from you, then slow it down and go lighter.

You should also try different positions for oral sex, and asking her what's best is always a good bet. If she's on her back, try slipping a pillow underneath her butt for an extra lift and to give you a better angle. When she's straddling your face, she can feel like she's not lying back passively but taking a more active role in her pleasure. Ultimately, you want to make sure you are in a position that doesn't have you straining your neck or other muscles. You want to be able to go the distance, not stop halfway

Expert Muff-Diving Secrets

- *Dive in:* nothing compares to your wild abandon; if you're not covered in girl juice, you're not doing it right.

- *Start slow:* take time with your tongue to cover every inch of her pussy.

- *Tease:* tease her with your lips and mouth till she's so excited, she'll grab you by the ears and beg you to dive in.

- *Add some suction:* don't limit yourself to licking—suck gently on her clit.

- *Mix it up:* side to side, up and down, circular, figure eights—see what works best for her.

through for a cramp. If you do get tired and need a break, take over with your hand, and alternate between hand and mouth. Remember that every woman's pussy is unique, as is the way she likes it licked. Women enjoy gentle licks, quick flicks of the tongue, clitoris sucking, noses pressing, and a bevy of other sensations you can create.

One more thing: every woman appreciates feeling a clean shave rub against their tender parts, rather than sandpaper stubble. Speaking of shaving, taking a razor to her pussy can not only be fun and erotic, but will heighten the sensations of oral sex. (Read more about shaving in the Q&A at the end of this chapter.)

Giving Great Head

There's no doubt about it: most men love a good blow job. Plenty of women aim to please in this department, but that usually requires patience and practice. In other words, women do not come out of the womb expert cocksuckers. Most guys will tell you that the more fun she's having with the rod, the better the experience for him.

It's always best to start out with the tease. Hold his cock in your hand, lick the head, and stimulate it with flicks of your tongue. Don't neglect his testicles, his perineum, and other sweet spots on his body while you're getting ready to take him in your mouth. Try opening your mouth and gently tapping his cock against your tongue; the visual alone will make him weak in the knees. Keep in mind that he doesn't necessarily have to be rock hard for you to begin a spirited blow job. Take him in your mouth and feel as he stiffens between your lips; it will turn both of you on. Begin by generously licking his shaft from top to bottom, covering all sides. This full-coverage mouth treatment teases him *and* lubes the pole, making it slick and much easier to slide right down. Once you're ready to begin sliding your mouth down his shaft, be mindful of your teeth (ouch!). Purse your lips into an O that covers them. And while you're pursing, you can also experiment with adding more pressure with your lips to increase the friction around his cock.

You ultimately want to achieve a smooth, single-motion slide that pays close attention to his sensitive head. Go slow at first, then vary your speed, seeing what his body responds to. You also want to play with the depth of penetration in your mouth. Lots of women feel nervous about taking a cock far enough into their mouths. Use your hand—there's no law against it, and your digits will help you cover more area than you can with just your mouth. Coordinate your rhythm, so that your mouth and hand work in tandem in one motion to create continuous friction and

Mastering the Art of the Blow Job

- *Get into it:* he likes it best when you're having the time of your life and demonstrating it by looking at him, talking dirty in between, or losing yourself in the act.

- *Relax your throat:* it's mind over matter, girls. Just take a deep breath and take as much as you feel comfortable. Use your hand to make up the rest of the length.

- *Purse those lips:* the pressure of your lips can create a pleasurable sensation of friction.

- *Hit the spot:* With his cock in your mouth, try pressing on his sensitive perineum or, if he's game, slip a lubed finger in his ass to stimulate his prostate.

motion. Sure, a no-handed blow job is certainly impressive, but more difficult to pull off without practice; it's a nice variation, but be very mindful of your teeth. If you wanna pull a "deep throat," it may be hard to sustain for more than a few good deep strokes, but throw it in at a few choice moments and you can really make it intense for him.

Try as they might, some women simply have trouble giving head because of their gag reflex. The more nervous or worried you are, the worse the tension in the back of your throat will be. In order to solve this common problem, try to concentrate on relaxing the back of your throat. If it's still too much to make giving head comfortable for you, use your hand and just concentrate your mouth on the head—it's the most sensitive part anyway. Guys, a word of advice to you: let her be in control of the action. You can touch her face while she's working her magic. It's also helpful to hear your comments, but most women are turned off when you grab their head and push them down there.

Don't Forget the Back Door

Anilingus, more commonly known as "rimming," is stimulation of the anal area with the mouth and tongue—licking, flicking, nibbling, sucking, circling, and tongue-fucking. Many people love the simple pleasure of having their ass licked or licking a partner's ass. Because the anal area is so full of nerve endings, even the tiniest sensations can register big on the turn-on meter. A good way to introduce rimming is to begin by nibbling and licking your partner's butt cheeks. As with other activities, it's important to explore and pleasure the whole area, rather than diving right into the crown jewel. Once you're ready to put your mouth on the anus, start out slowly. Explore every little nook of your lover's asshole—there are a million little folds and crevices to find and lick.

Some people may feel especially anxious about rimming because of the association between the asshole and defecating; we learn at an early age that if something is dirty or smells bad, we shouldn't put our mouth on it. Remember that there are normally no feces in the anus and anal canal. With proper bowel movements and regular hygiene, the anus is almost as clean as the vagina, which many of us lick with desire and enthusiasm. However, the bacteria in our rectum and feces can cause gastrointestinal problems, so use common sense.

Let your lips and tongue explore your lover's ass freely and experiment with different techniques as you go along. Listen to your partner's verbal and nonverbal responses and let those help guide you. Some people like to really thrust their tongues in and out of their partner's anus; you can penetrate and fuck your lover's ass to ecstasy.

Q&A

I *told my boyfriend that I was going to shave my pussy, and he says he'd like to do it. Do you have any tips for us before I go under the blade?*

Both women and men like to groom their pubic hair; I think it's absolutely healthy, and a sex therapist once told me that women who regularly clip or shave their pubes have a better relationship with their pussies since they make time to look at them in a mirror and fuss over them while primping. Shaving can be practical, but it can also be an erotic activity in and of itself, whether you do it alone or with a partner. I absolutely feel sexier after I have shaved my own pussy; once all the hair comes off, I can see every inch and every fold of my own genitals. The area is also left unprotected and I become hyperaware of what's between my legs when I walk, sit down, or make any kind of move. Entrusting someone else to take a very sharp object to a very tender spot can be scary, exciting, and awfully arousing.

I do have some practical advice for you. If you have never trimmed any of that hair before, it's a good idea to start out with clippers or a pair of scissors to trim it down to a more manageable bush. Before you shave, begin by gently exfoliating the skin with a soft brush (like a face brush or even a vegetable brush) and a fragrance-free exfoliating scrub. Of course, when shaving yourself or another person, you should do it in a clean, well-lit place, go slow, and be careful. Lather the area with a good shaving cream or gel, preferably one with no dyes or scents that could irritate your delicate vagina. Use a good, sharp razor (leave the wielding of straight razors to the professionals!); I prefer one of the newer models with a triple blade (such as Gillette Mach 3) over the cheap disposable single-blade kind.

Begin with the pubic mound and work your way down to the more tender parts. Shave with, rather than against, the grain. If you need to, pull the skin taut to prevent nicks or scrapes. Rinse the area with cool water. It's probably not a good idea to shave the area right before you're planning to have sex. It may become more easily irritated, and a cut might provide an opportunity for STD transmission. When the hair grows back, it will itch, so use a soothing lotion. However, I find that the more frequently you shave, the less it itches as long as you keep up with it.

If you're looking for other ways to simply remove the hair, some women do have their bikini line and beyond waxed. Waxing is a lot messier and definitely more painful. While I know some folks who do their own waxing at home, I say leave it to the professionals. Unless you've experienced another part of your body being waxed, I would not recommend that your first waxing experience be with your tender genitals. All I can say is "Ouch!" I suggest you first get some other part of your body waxed to see if you want to use that particular method on your private parts. Skip creams like Nair that promise to "remove hair"; they shouldn't be used in the genital area. If you are wondering about electrolysis, it can been done safely and effectively. There is a certain amount of pain with any electrolysis (some people describe it as a slight needle prick or a quick burning sensation), and I think that because your genital area is sensitive to begin with, there's probably more pain than, say, having your legs done. Electrolysis is permanent, although only after several treatments (about four or five), and it is expensive. It's an investment in time and money, and if I were you, I would definitely do some research into a good dermatologist or cosmetologist to do the procedure. Oh, and all these methods can also be applied to shaving your ass, or shaving a man's balls and pubic area. Turnabout is fair play, after all.

4

WHAT YOU NEED TO GET THE JOB DONE

Sex Tools and Sex Toys

There was a time when many believed that all you had to do to have great sex was put two naked people in a room together and let nature take its course. When adult novelties were gag gifts you giggled over at bachelor parties. When the only time you saw a dildo was in a porno. When vibrators and other sex toys were called "marital aids." That time has passed. There is a wide world of products out there designed with one purpose in mind—to make your sex life better. If you want to have the very best sex of your life, you need to take advantage of all the available tools for the job. Some people still believe that lubricants, vibrators, and other toys are for losers without lovers, couples with sexual problems, or people who can't get the job done with their God-given parts. I like to think of it as just the opposite. Some of the most sexually active and adventurous men and women regularly use all sorts of tools to kick their sex lives up a notch. Incorporating erotic products into your lovemaking routines can change your sexual world. Explore desires and fantasies you never knew you had. Transform a cuddly quickie into an all-night affair. Turn the everyday bump and grind into extraordinary sex. Make a one-come girl into a multiorgasmic woman.

Lubricants

Personal lubricants have been around for a long time, and before K-Y jelly was first introduced, I am sure people were improvising. When AIDS became an epidemic in the United States, sex educators were encouraging people to use latex condoms, gloves, and dental dams to protect themselves. With a lubricant, latex is much less likely to break; inside and outside a condom, lube increases movement, sensitivity, and pleasure. Thus, latex and lube were perfect partners in the safer sex revolution. As a result of the increase in safer sex practices, the use of lube rose in popularity, and there are now more brands available than ever before. But with or without latex, I think lube makes every kind of sex better; after all, the wetter and more slippery all the parts get, the hotter everything else gets, right? Doesn't everyone want a slicker hand job, a juicier finger fuck, a smoother rear entry, and even a moister muff dive? Of course you do! I am still perplexed that there isn't a tube, bottle, or supersize pump of lube on every bedside table in America, but I am hoping to change that.

Many men resist using lube during sex because they feel threatened by anything they perceive as a sexual helper. When a customer at Toys in Babeland chose to buy his wife a sizable vibrator, I suggested he also purchase some lube. He declined, insisting, "Oh, we don't need that. I can turn her on all by myself." This is a common exchange. I tried to persuade him gently, when what I really wanted to say was: the fact of the matter is that she may be plenty turned on, but that doesn't mean she'll be slick enough to take that big vibe with ease. If she's not comfortable, chances are her pleasure will be compromised. Get over your insecurities and get some lube in your life!

Women too are often embarrassed or feel insecure about using a lubricant. We need to assure ourselves that using lube does not mean there is something wrong with us. In the mainstream media, lube is marketed only to postmenopausal women, since many experience vaginal dryness during and after menopause. But lube is for women of all ages.

Women are blessed with vaginas that naturally lubricate when they become aroused. But the truth is that some women are just wetter than others. For many women, how much they lubricate is not based on desire alone. There are many factors that affect how much or little women's vaginas lubricate, including menstrual cycle, pregnancy, breast-feeding, recent surgery, diet, general health, dehydration, exercise, stress level, medications, and others. In other words, you could be totally aroused, but still experience vaginal dryness.

A little lube is all you need to make penetration smoother and easier, which will leave you feeling more relaxed and sexy in the long run. Many women still silently endure friction (not the good kind), irritation, and pain from penetration that could easily be rectified by using proper lubrication. And if your partner has a larger than usual basket, well, good for him, but maybe not so good for you. Lube will help you make good use of the average to the ample, rather than leaving you feeling overwhelmed and impaled. As for anal penetration, well, you simply cannot do it without lube. And men, we know that a hand job, yours or hers, can always be improved with lube.

You may be considering (or actually using) some common household items as lube. Many people use vegetable oil, Vaseline, baby oil, lotion, or moisturizer. While they may grease the pole, these substances are not meant to be used for sex, so they don't have any of the outstanding properties of sexual lubricants. They don't stay wet for very long. Because they are oil-based, they also break down latex, so are not compatible with condoms or gloves. They are just not as good as lubes that were researched, developed, and tested especially for sex. But most important, oil-based lubricants like those mentioned are impossible to wash out of the vagina; they are a breeding ground for bacteria and very likely to cause an infection. A woman in one of my workshops asked what she could do to give her husband a really good hand job. "We use lotion, but it dries pretty quickly," she said. Not only will lube work better, but it's safer for him to fuck her after she works him with her hand without the risk of sticking lotion in her pussy where it doesn't belong. Men, if you are married to that Vaseline for a hand job, make sure you wipe, then wash your penis off before you put it inside her vagina. As for anal penetration, the rectum naturally flushes itself out, so there is less, but still some, risk of infection. If you use an oil-based lubricant in a woman's ass, it is very difficult to keep a small amount of that lube from dripping, migrating, or otherwise finding its way into the vagina. So, in general, you should leave oil-based lubes in the kitchen and bathroom where they belong.

Now let me address that old gooey standard, K-Y jelly. Here are the best things K-Y has going for it: you can find it in any drugstore in America (and maybe even the in-laws' medicine cabinet) and it will do in a pinch. But K-Y was designed for brief medical exams, not a rockin' carnal marathon, if you know what I mean. K-Y does make a lubricant marketed for "intimacy" (I just love their discretion) called K-Y Liquid which is better than its forefather the jelly. So, just put that K-Y jelly in your natural-disaster emergency kit along with the flashlight and canned food and move into the new millennium where there are many different kinds of water-based and silicone-based lubricants designed especially for sex.

Nonstaining, easy to clean up, and available in a variety of textures, water-based lubricants are condom-compatible and safe to use. Made with many different ingredients, the main one in most water-based lubes is glycerin, which gives it the ability to stay slick during sex. Some lubricants have a slight taste—either sweet, slightly chemical, or even bitter—and others don't. The rule of thumb (and forefinger) with lube is to try several differ-ent brands. What lube is the *best* lube? The one that works for you. Better sex-toy stores sell sample-size packets of lube, and I encourage you to buy several different kinds, try them out, and then pick your favorite.

Thin, liquidy lubes feel most like women's natural vaginal flu-ids, which make them great for vaginal penetration. Brand names include Astroglide, Eros Woman Water Formulation, K-Y Liquid, Foreplay Lube de Luxe Liquid, Probe Light, and Wet Light. There are also thicker lubes, with consistencies like hair gel or even Vaseline. Thicker lubes tend to stay wet longer, so you have to reapply them less often. Because you need plenty of lubrication, thick lubes are a better choice than their thinner counterparts for anal penetration. Because of their gel-like qual-ities, they have a cushioning effect inside the delicate lining of the rectum that can make anal penetration easier and more comfortable. Examples of thick lubes are ID, Foreplay Lube de Luxe Gel or Cream, Foreplay Original, Probe Thick, and Wet Original.

If you are particularly sensitive to glycerin (and many women are) or allergic to it, you should choose a water-based glycerin-free lube. Liquid Silk and Slippery Stuff Liquid are thinner, while Hydra-Smooth, Maximus, and Slippery Stuff Gel are thicker. Glycerin-free lubes tend to dry up more quickly than those with glycerin, so either rehydrate them with a little bit of water or add more lube as needed. Glycerin-free water-based lubes are also a smart choice for women who are especially prone to chronic yeast, urinary tract, or other vaginal infections. Women who are sensitive or allergic to glycerin or prone to infections should also definitely avoid flavored lubricants. It might be a good idea for most women to avoid using flavored lubricants for penetration, and reserve them just for fellatio. I am not a big fan of flavored lubes because my feeling is that I'd like to experience how my partner tastes rather than cover it up with some mouthwashy mint or artificially-flavored strawberry.

However, if you are practicing safer sex and using oral barriers for cunnilingus, analingus, and fellatio, the taste of latex can be less than ideal. In those cases, a flavored lube might help you forget your mouth is on rubber and facilitate the task at hand—getting your partner to a state of ecstasy! ID Juicy Lube comes in several flavors, as do Foreplay Succulents and Wet Flavored Lubricants; check ingredients very carefully, since some of these fruity lubes may contain sugar or artificial sugar substitutes which are more likely to cause a yeast infection or aggravate a chronic yeast imbalance.

Silicone-based lubricants are the newest on the market; they are nontoxic and feel extremely light and slick to the touch. These lubes boast that they'll give you the most slippery ride of your life, and it's true—lubes made of silicone stay wet for a very long time. Depending on the brand and its ingredients (read those labels, folks!), silicone lubes may or may not be tasteless and odorless. Because of its unique properties, silicone does not get sticky or tacky like a water-based lube. Many people report that silicone lubes are so thin, that you barely feel them. Their slickness make penetration smoother and easier while still allowing for plenty of pleasurable friction.

However, silicone is not absorbed into the body's skin or tissue like water-based and oil-based lubes, which is why it stays slick forever, even longer than you may want it to. Because you can't wash silicone out of your body, you have to wait for the body to naturally flush the lube out; this process obviously happens faster in your rectum than in your vagina. If the lube is made of pure silicone without added sugar or other ingredients, there is no danger of a bacterial infection since silicone is a completely inert substance; check the ingredients since each brand is different. Wet International, maker of Wet Platinum silicone lube, also sells a product called Lubricant After Wash that helps to "degrease" you after sex with a silicone lube.

Silicone-based lubes are completely safe to use with latex and condoms. However, in some cases, silicone has a chemical reac-

Lubes at a Glance

Water-Based Lubes That Contain Glycerin

BRANDS: Astroglide, Eros Water Formulation, K-Y, Foreplay, ID, Sex Grease, Wet

PRO: easy to clean up, variety of textures, nonstaining, latex compatible, some available in flavors

CON: glycerin may cause yeast infections in some women

TIP: add a little water to revive when it dries up

Water-Based Lubes Without Glycerin

BRANDS: Hydra Smooth, Liquid Silk, Maximus, Slippery Stuff

PRO: less likely to cause or aggravate yeast infections and other chemical sensitivities; latex compatible

CON: Because they do not contain glycerin, these lubes tend to dry up much faster, and you need to re-lube more frequently.

TIP: best for women who've experienced sensitivity to other lubes or chronic yeast infections

"Natural" Lubes (Water-Based)

BRANDS: O'My, Probe, Sylk

PRO: contain natural ingredients like grapefruit seed extract, hemp, kiwi, aloe; latex compatible

CON: may not have the long-lasting properties of lubes with artificial ingredients

TIP: Read the labels carefully; even natural ingredients may irritate some women.

Silicone-Based Lubes

BRANDS: Eros, Eros Woman, ID Millennium, Wet Platinum

PRO: stay wet for a very long time; latex compatible

CON: never wash out; incompatible with some silicone toys

TIP: Try Wet's After Wash for easier cleanup.

Oil-Based Lubes

BRANDS: Vaseline, baby oil, Crisco, Wesson, various lotions

PRO: inexpensive, easy to find

CON: don't wash out; can cause vaginal infections; break down latex

TIP: Don't use them for sex.

tion when it comes into contact with another silicone; this means that silicone lubricants can ruin some silicone sex toys (including dildos, butt plugs, and vibrators). If you want to use a silicone lube with a silicone toy, use a condom to protect the toy from being damaged. Silicone lubes are more expensive than water-based lubes, yet some people would argue that the cost ends up being the same since you use much less silicone lube.

Depending on the brand and its ingredients, lube can feel like WD-40, liquid soap, lotion, hair gel, or petroleum jelly. You should always pour lube into your hand and spread it around with your fingers or onto a cock or sex toy. Never pour it directly into any orifice. Start out with a small handful, and add more if and when you need it. If you are using a water-based lube, eventually it will start to dry up, becoming sticky and tacky. You have two options: you can add a little water to it, which will "revive" the lube, making it slick and wet again, or simply add more lube. Inside you, lube should feel wet and wonderful; it should not itch, burn, or otherwise feel irritating. If it does, you are most likely sensitive or allergic to it. Rinse the lube out with warm water and a little soap as best you can. Next time, try a different brand and see if that works better for you.

To give him a slick hand job, pour some lube into your hand

and coat his cock from base to head. The lube will make your hand slide smoothly and easily up and down. When it loses its slickness and starts to get sticky, add a little water or some more lube. Especially if you are using a condom, but even if you are not, try lubing his shaft and head before you give him a blow job. Use your finger to trace your lips with lube (this is when flavor or an inoffensive taste is essential), then slide them down his shaft in one effortless stroke.

To rub her the right way, lube up your fingers and gently spread it around her pussy. Stroke her lips and the opening of her vagina. Work your way up to her clit, then rub her clitoris just the way she likes it. If her clit starts to dry up, try dipping your fingers inside her and reviving the lube with her natural wetness. Whether you've got a barrier or not, lubing her pussy before your mouth goes down there will make your job easier and enhance her enjoyment of your hard work. Choose a lube with a taste you like (you could pick a flavored one, but why mask her luscious taste?), and happy diving!

Fingers, penises, and sex toys will slide inside smoother and easier with some lube. You can introduce the slippery stuff in a way that makes it fun and sexy, rather than an unnatural interruption of the, um, flow of things. Lube should come onto the scene sooner rather than later. In other words, waiting until intercourse isn't the best use of it. For women, introducing lube early in foreplay starts to get the juices flowing. It feels good, so it will enhance her pleasure no matter what you're doing to her. It may also put her mind and body at ease if she usually feels pressure to get wet quickly.

For example, you can give him a hand job with lube, and when you're ready to have him inside you, give him some extra grease and climb on! Guys, you may want to take a handful of lube and masturbate for her. Your cock will be well lubricated, and she will have gotten a sexy little show. The same goes for the girls—you can masturbate for him, getting your pussy nice and slick with lube while you tempt him with what's just around the corner. If the foreplay is extensive (which, by the way, I always recommend!), make sure to re-lube everything before penetration. Lube makes each rub, each stroke, each thrust smoother, more comfortable, and potentially more pleasurable for both partners, no matter what the activity.

The Sex-Toy Revolution

Once an industry that focused on adult novelties designed for humor rather than function, sex-toy manufacturing has radically changed. Bachelor-party jokes and cheap, badly designed devices are still around, but many companies have an entirely different vision of adult products. Though still primarily in the novelty biz, industry veterans like Doc Johnson and California Exotics/Swedish Erotica have been making rubber dongs for a long, long time. The plus of these traditionalists is that they are well distributed and can be found in adult book and video stores nationwide. Plus, these companies have changed with the times and added some sophisticated products to go with their trashy blowup dolls. Armed with market research, product testing, and a sex-positive attitude, smaller, less well-known companies are making tools that not only work and are safe, but bring pleasure to thousands of people every year.

Once upon a time, the only place you could find a dildo was at a sleazy adult book or video store, squeezed in a small glass case all the way in the back. There is a whole new breed of sex-toy shops around the country, places like Toys in Babeland in Seattle and New York, Grand Opening outside Boston, A Woman's Touch in Madison, and Good Vibrations in San Francisco. (See the Resource Guide at the end of the book for more information.) These clean, well-lit, sex-positive places have friendly and extremely knowledgeable salespeople who sell high-quality products and encourage their customers to explore and be empowered by sex. I urge you to take a trip to the store near you or order a catalog; these are truly revolutionary places that can change your sex life! The great thing about actually going to the store (rather than ordering online or through the mail) is that you can see and feel all the products. Plus, you can talk to the people who work there, who are experienced and knowledgeable.

Here's a look at a variety of vibrators, cock rings, and dildos to give you some ideas about what's out there. (I will cover all anal-sex toys, including butt plugs and anal beads, in chapter 6.)

The Joy of Vibrators

There's a reason that hotels catering to lunchtime quickies and sex workers have vibrating beds. There's a reason some women like to ride motorcycles and others like to sit on the drier while their sheets are fluffing dry. Both relaxing and stimulating, vibration is a wonderful addition to any sex life. Like people, vibrators come in all shapes and sizes, all speeds and styles, and some even come with attachments! Whether electric or battery-operated, these sex toys deliver a buzzing vibration that sends most women (and plenty of men) over the moon. The information in this section will focus on vibrators for women; however, you guys will get some buzz time at the end. While different vibrators produce different sensations, the feeling of a vibrator is unmatched—they move faster than any tongue or hand ever can. They also deliver a more consistent movement than any human being, and their reliability during solo or partner sex is unmatched. For some people, vibrators deliver a much stronger sensation than they can produce with their own hand or their partner's.

Before I went to work at Toys in Babeland, I had owned and used one vibrator pretty sporadically. I guess being surrounded by the best and brightest inspired me; plus, how could I honestly recommend our products if I hadn't tried them myself? So, I purchased several different models and took them home for a test drive. Here I am, several vibes and dozens of batteries later, and I am hooked! What is most appealing is their power and consistency—they never get tired, uncomfortable, or lazy like my own hand does. And using them with a partner means I can concentrate on other things.

Designed for external use, internal use, or both, vibrators are especially outstanding for clitoral stimulation. They are often recommended for women who've never had an orgasm or who have a hard time achieving one. If this describes you, I definitely encourage you to try a vibrator. Dr. Betty Dodson, masturbation guru and author of *Sex for One*, swears by vibrators for helping women come, come longer, come faster, and come better!

Selecting a Vibrator

When choosing a vibrator—especially if it's your first one—I absolutely recommend a trip to the sex-toy store. You can see them in the (fake) flesh, pick them up, turn them on, feel the vibration, listen to the noise they make, and see what might work best for you. Your first consideration should be power: do you want a vibration that moves you gently to orgasm or do you need one that can shake the whole room? In general, plug-in vibrators are much more powerful than their battery-operated counterparts. But electricity also means access to a plug, so you need to be relatively close to an outlet or an extension cord. You've got to sacrifice convenience for strength. Most plug-in models, marketed in mainstream stores and catalogs as "personal massagers," should be used for external stimulation only. If it's really reliable, potent clitoral stimulation you're after, then a plug-in vibrator is best for you. Battery-operated vibrators usually require AA or C batteries. Some vibes have a separate battery pack, attached with a cord, with on/off and speed controls, while others are one unit. Some vibrators have two (or more) speeds, while others have a dial that lets you vary the speed. If you are intimidated by the drill-like speed of a plug-in or think you need only a moderate amount of vibration to get you off, then a battery-operated vibrator should be just fine. Sound may also be a consideration, especially if you have kids, roommates, thin walls, or nosy neighbors. That's another reason why testing them out is a good idea.

Your next question should be: what do I want my vibrator to do? Remember, all vibrators can be used externally to stimulate the clitoris and the other areas of the vagina. Some models (especially the plug-in variety) can only be used on the outside of the body. Other vibrators are designed for penetration. There is also a line of dual-action vibrators that are multitasking gems; the best are manufactured and imported from Japan, but there are some less expensive American knockoffs. Dual-action vibrators are made for *simultaneous* penetration and clitoral stimulation.

Most plug-ins are made of plastic or a combination of plastic and rubber. Battery-operated vibes range from hard plastic to soft jelly or firmer rubber. There are a select few made of silicone, which is the ideal sex-toy material. Silicone is super easy to clean (see "Care and Cleaning of Vibrators" at the end of this section), warms up with use and retains body heat, and is much more resilient than rubber.

Your personal taste will also figure into your selection—how do you want your vibrator to look? The majority of battery-operated vibes are phallic. Some simply mimic the shape of a penis, without an exact representation, while others are made to look more realistic. They come in all sorts of colors, from so-called flesh tones to rainbow brights; fancier models have flowers, animal prints, or even glittery sparkles. Most electric models look like ordinary massagers and may or may not come with an assortment of attachments. The nonphallic battery-operated ones are shaped like bullets, eggs, or cute animals (again courtesy of the Japanese). Some women are turned off by a slightly garish hot pink sparkly cock and want a more innocuous-looking object that looks less like a sex toy. Others don't mind a

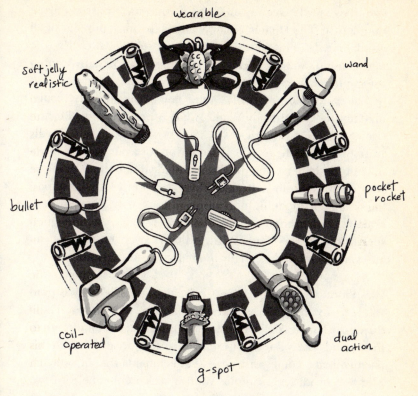

wearable

soft jelly realistic

wand

bullet

pocket rocket

coil-operated

g-spot

dual action

FIG. 5   VIBRATORS

little glitter if it gets the job done. It's totally up to you. The following are some popular models you may want to consider. (Also see illustration 5.)

Popular Vibrator Models

Wand Vibrators (plug-in, $40–68): Electric wand vibrators are the most powerful and the largest of the pack, usually nearly a foot long with a large round head. As you can imagine, these are meant for external, clitoral stimulation only. Because of their size, they may be slightly awkward if you want to use it during intercourse. The Hitachi Magic Wand is the most popular of all wand models. Thousands of women absolutely swear by the Magic Wand, and for them nothing else will do. Many women who've never used or owned a vibrator used to come into Toys in Babeland asking for the Wand and saying friends recommended it. The Hitachi Magic Wand is probably not the best choice for a first vibrator. It's just too powerful and can actually scare women off from ever using a vibrator again if their introduction to them is something that could vibrate the enamel off your teeth. Not only it is super-strong and pretty loud, its imposing size alone might intimidate the first-time user. There are several plastic attachments (including a G-spot one) designed specifically for the Magic Wand which fit over the round head and can be inserted vaginally or anally.

Coil Vibrators (plug-in, $32–36): Smaller and slightly less powerful than wands, coil vibrators are strong, quiet types. These sturdy workhorses deliver a more focused, speedy vibration than their wand sisters due to the smaller surface area of their head. Each coil vibe comes with several attachments that fit over the vibrating head; for example, Wahl makes a coil vibe with two speeds and seven different attachments. Plus, there are other attachments created especially for coil vibrators and sold separately, some of which can turn this external-stimulation-only vibe into one for penetration, too.

Pocket Rocket (battery operated, $20–24): Only a little bigger than a lipstick and powered by one battery, the Pocket Rocket is one of the best battery-operated vibrators on the market. Designed for clitoral stimulation, this two-speed jewel (which also comes in a waterproof model) can literally fit in your pocket and packs a powerful punch. You can bring it anywhere—keep one in the glove compartment for the dreaded commute, one in your desk drawer at work to relieve stress on the job. With its innocuous look, even the most timid of women will warm up to this baby. The Pocket Rocket is perfect for adding clitoral stimulation to vaginal or anal penetration with a partner because its compact size won't get in the way.

Slimline or Smoothie (battery operated, $10–20): The most traditional of all vibrators, the hard plastic vibrator looks like the giant top of a lipstick. Smooth, slick, and available in a variety of colors, the Slimline is economical and gets the job done. It comes in a variety of lengths and widths, but the most widely available size doesn't really live up to its name (about 6½ inches long and 1¼ inches in diameter). While its phallic shape makes one automatically think of penetration, its hard exterior suggests a poke in the pussy. Penetration with a Slimline is only good for gals who prefer something very solid—its hard, inflexible plastic is definitely not everyone's cup of tea. I think this vibe is often overlooked because it looks cheap and the price tag matches. The truth is that for external stimulation, its variable speed is powerful enough to suit most women and its size promises that it will cover enough surface area. This vibrator can be more difficult to use with a partner, but not impossible, especially if you're in doggie-style position.

Soft Rubber and Jelly Vibes (battery operated, $12–25): These are the most common generic vibes on the market, and the easiest to find (most often in realistic penis styles). A word of caution: they can really vary in power, speed, and noise level and are not made to stand the test of time. A relatively low vibration rarely makes them good for clitoral stimulation; however, they are made of a softer rubber which many women find more comfortable and pleasurable for penetration. But definitely use plenty of lube. Newer models also incorporate a curved shape, some more exaggerated than others, to hit the G-spot.

Pros and Cons of Popular Vibrators

Hitachi Magic Wand

POWER: plug-in
LOOK: like a portable blender
PRO: the most powerful vibration
CON: its size could intimidate a first-timer
TIP: Use a washcloth to muffle and lessen the vibration if it's too strong for you.

Wahl Seven-in-One

POWER: plug-in
LOOK: like a mixer, without the egg-beater attachments
PRO: strong and fairly quiet
CON: not exactly compact, awkward for partner sex
TIP: Try all the different attachments.

Pocket Rocket

POWER: battery
LOOK: a super-compact massager
PRO: small size, discreet look, pretty powerful
CON: Not as powerful as plug-in; quality varies between different brands
TIP: Use the waterproof version in the shower or anywhere else wet.

Slimline (a.k.a. Smoothie)

POWER: battery
LOOK: a giant, extra-long lipstick top
PRO: inexpensive, covers lots of surface area, power varies by model

CON: can be too hard and pointy for pleasurable penetration
TIP: Position it between your legs lengthwise—one end works your
clit, the other slips between your lips for extra stimulation.

Jelly Vibe

POWER: battery
LOOK: fake plastic penis, ranging from slightly silly to hideous
PRO: inexpensive, widely available
CON: vibration may be too mild for most clits, better for penetration
TIP: Use a condom on this one to get the most use out of it and
make it easier to clean.

Dual-Action

POWER: battery
LOOK: carved totem pole with animal attachment
PRO: simultaneous clit stimulation, vaginal stimulation and penetration
CON: expensive, potential for overstimulation
TIP: Start with only one feature on to warm up, then add the others.

Natural Contours

POWER: battery
LOOK: modern, streamlined
PRO: discreet looking and well constructed
CON: highest vibration can be pretty tame for some women
TIP: Take advantage of its curved shape: slip it inside your panties,
turn over on your stomach, and ride into the sunset.

Pros and Cons of Popular Vibrators *(Continued)*

Wearable

POWER: battery
LOOK: friendly little animal, looks like a gummi bear
PRO: designed to wear during intercourse
CON: straps can tangle easily, vibe can slip around and may have to be held in place, defeating its wearable design
TIP: Keep the controls handy so you can adjust the speed without breaking away from the position you're in.

Dual-Action Vibrators (battery operated, $50–120): The Japanese make some of the finest sex toys available today, and they have the market cornered on the dual-action vibrator. Sure, there are plenty of American knockoffs of this product, but they simply cannot compare to the original. The idea behind the dual action is to provide stimulation right inside the vaginal opening, vaginal penetration, and clitoral stimulation simultaneously. A rubber, phallic vibrating dildo is coupled with a cute vibrating animal whose ears, tongue, or nose works your clit. The Japanese are especially fond of incorporating little critters into their sex toys. Depending on the model, the vibrating dildo part cannot only vibrate, but rotate in one or both directions. Some of these vibrators contain a ring in the dildo filled with beads which dance around (think of a Lotto machine with its numbered balls); the ring is meant to hit just inside the vaginal opening—the most sensitive part of the vagina for many women—for an extra sensation. The dildo part and the clit part have separate controls, with a myriad of possibilities. You can put the dildo inside without vibration, rotation, or beads and just the clitoral vibe on. You can start with the dildo vibrating to warm up then add the clit crit. Or you can have it all at once. These are the most expensive vibrators on the market, so beginners may want to try some of the simpler battery-operated vibes before making a serious investment in a dual-action vibrator.

Natural Contours (battery operated, $35–40): Designed by feminist porn producer Candida Royalle, these well-constructed, hard plastic vibrators come in several different sizes and are made for external stimulation only. Nonphallic, with a modern, streamlined curved design, they are among the most discreet looking of all vibrators. If you are concerned about someone discovering your little pet or are simply turned off by the traditional phallic shape of many vibrators, then this is the one for you. Its vibration, with three variable speeds, is mild to moderate compared to others. If you are looking for a nonintimidating vibe designed by a woman, Natural Contours is a great choice.

Wearable Vibrators (battery operated, $22–38): There are tiny but powerful vibrators that come with adjustable elastic leg straps; you can actually strap the vibe onto your body and position it exactly where you want it for hands-free fun. They usually take the form of cutesy butterflies, ladybugs, and dolphins, but don't let that dissuade you. They really work and tend to be among the quieter vibes. Many women find that these are ideal for use during vaginal intercourse since their size means they don't get in the way of penetration and don't require some advanced Twister moves to hold the thing in place. But depending on how tight you wear it and how much you move around, you may have to hold it in place with a finger or two. In missionary position especially, you can be face-to-face with your partner while the little critter does all the work! Some stores also sell a leather panty with leg straps and a pouch for a small vibrator to be tucked in. Vibrating eggs or bullet-shaped vibes with a separate battery pack work best. Some women find that leather feels better than plastic, the panty actually muffles the sound of the vibration, and they can experiment with different vibrating eggs without buying a whole new apparatus. To get the most powerful one of these little critters, look for one that takes three or more batteries.

Using a Vibrator

If you've never used a vibrator before, you should start out with a simple one that has variable speeds so you can experiment with what works best for you. I also recommend that you choose one with a moderate speed. Vibrators take some getting used to, and chances are if you've never had one on your clit, a moderate one will be just fine. If you get used to it and find you want more juice, you can always upgrade later. If you are hesitant at all about a vibrator, choose one of the nonintimidating, quiet models so you can ease your way into it.

Many women like to use a vibrator alone while masturbating, which is a great road to self-pleasure and orgasm. It's also a perfect way to work out the kinks and decide what you like (which you may want to share with your partner later). Begin by turning the vibrator to its lowest setting; use it to stimulate your labia, the opening of your vagina, and the perineum. Move it around and explore what feels good; you can also experiment with different levels of pressure and see how different speeds feel. As you become more aroused, place the vibrator above or to one side of your clitoral hood. This indirect approach will help you get used to the buzzing sensation. For some women, a vibrator near the clitoral hood is enough to start their body humming and even achieve orgasm. If you want to feel more direct stimulation, place the vibrator directly on the clitoral hood. This will feel a lot more intense; if it feels too intense, back off on the pressure, decrease the speed, or move it back to the side. Make sure you are turned on before you put a vibe right on the clitoral hood; in a nonaroused state, your clit will most likely feel too sensitive to handle a vibrator right away. I know some women who actually pull back the clitoral hood and go right for the glans, and you may want to try that when you're pretty turned on—for others, it's way too sensitive to do that.

Once you find a comfortable position for the vibrator, a good speed, and the right amount of pressure, begin to explore some different kinds of movement. Some women like to move the vibrator up and down or side to side; others will actually hold the vibe still and move themselves on top of it. If your vibrator is made for penetrating, you can put it inside and add another vibe for clit stimulation or alternate between the two. If you want more of an indirect vibration, you can put the vibrator against your hand and your hand against your clit.

If you find that the vibration feels overwhelming or too intense, you have a few options. You may have purchased too powerful a vibrator and you're going to have to get another one with less power. But sometimes yesterday's perfect buzz seems way too strong today. Our bodies change with our menstrual cycles, stress, diet, exercise, and illness, and sometimes we just feel more physically sensitive. In that case, I recommend turning the vibrator down or putting a few fingers between your clit and your buzzing friend. You may also simply need to work your way up to the strong vibration. One trick I learned from Betty Dodson, the mother of masturbation, is to put a washcloth between the vibrator and your clit. You can fold the washcloth as many times as you need to, and it will act as a buffer to lessen the vibration. Gradually, as you get more practice and feel ready for stronger vibration, you can unfold the washcloth, making the barrier thinner and thinner until you no longer need it at all.

Using a Vibrator with Your Partner

In addition to gaining knowledge about your body and its pleasure, a wonderful result of experimenting with a vibrator by yourself is that you can dole out instructions to your partner about what feels good. That's right: vibrators aren't just for lonely spinsters, single gals, or those of you married to traveling salesmen. They can also be used as a fun addition to sex with your partner. Some men won't want their partners to use a vibrator for fear that it will replace them. The truth is that vibrators offer a unique sensation different from what a person can give you. But that doesn't mean that it renders people obsolete.

Men, you can discover a lot from watching a woman use her vibrator; learn how she masturbates with it, what feels good, how much pressure she likes, her unique sweet spots for clitoral stimulation. Vibrators can be a part of foreplay; your partner can use one to tease you and turn you on. Men, remember not to go directly for her clit with a vibe before she's had some warm-up with your hand or mouth first. Test the waters by exploring all different areas of her pussy with the vibrator. Depending on the type of vibrator, you can experiment with its possibilities. Vary the speed, pressure, and position of the vibe—she'll let you know when you've struck gold. Once she's worked up, she may want you to stop wandering around with it and stay in one place for a while, so be prepared to stop dawdling and get down to business.

Vibrators can help men be in two places at once when women use them to add clitoral stimulation to vaginal or anal penetration. Sometimes, you can be in a position ideal for thrusting and pumping, but one that doesn't lend itself to you working her clitoris. Okay, so you're not actually in two places at the same time, but all she will know is that your cock inside her feels even better with something buzzing against her clit. Models especially good for use during penetration with a partner are the ones that actually strap to the body, small models like the Pocket Rocket, and vibrating eggs that can be held in place with a couple of fingers. Depending on the position you are in, it might be most feasible for her to hold the vibe. In order to stay connected to her, put your hand over hers or reach for the

Care and Cleaning of Vibrators

Storage: Always store in a cool, dry place. You should remove the batteries from your vibrator when you're not using it to decrease the risk of accidental turn-on, which will run batteries down and may burn out your motor. This also prevents batteries from leaking or exploding inside your vibrator and damaging it.

Batteries: Many people in the sex industry recommend using Energizer batteries; through trial and error and lots of customer feedback, we've found that they seem to work the best. Duracell batteries, for whatever reasons, have been known to burn out the motors of different kinds of vibrators.

Cleaning: You should always unplug a vibrator or take out the batteries before you clean it and while you let it dry. Whether it plugs into the wall or is battery-operated, a vibrator should never be submerged in water—unless, of course, it is waterproof. Plug-in models should be wiped with a damp, soapy cloth, then again with a plain damp cloth. Vibrators made of hard plastic, rubber, or silicone can also be cleaned in the same fashion. Silicone vibrators are nonporous, but others are not. If you plan to share a vibrator, always use a condom on it.

vibrator and press it against her at an appropriate moment. You may want to consider using a vibrator for penetration in order to achieve double penetration with a partner; he may enjoy feeling the vibration while he is inside you.

Vibrators also come in handy when you and your partner want assistance for one reason or another. For example, maybe you've made a valiant effort to go down on her or give her an extended hand job. Your mouth or hand (or both) are tired, but she still wants to come, and she knows just the thing that will get her there—the vibrator. When she finally goes over the edge, you can still take credit for it, since your efforts made the relief pitcher's job that much easier.

Perhaps you shot your load before she did. She's still hot and heavy, but you are spent and sleepy. Reach for the vibrator, and you are back in action! Whether she wants more in-and-out or clitoral stimulation or both, you're now equipped to give her an orgasm as great as the one you just had.

If your gal is a multiorgasmic wonder and you're having trouble keeping up, a vibrator can be the solution, and your new best friend. It can keep her coming and coming as much as she likes, while keeping you from developing lockjaw or carpal tunnel syndrome. As long as you stay connected to her—instead of plugging the vibrator in and heading to the kitchen for a snack—vibrator sex can still be a two-person project that's just as fulfilling and satisfying as the old-fashioned way.

Vibrator Addiction?

Some women believe that they will become addicted to or reliant on a vibrator in order to achieve orgasm, and, unfortunately, this keeps them from ever trying one in the first place. Realize that most women find that the kind of orgasm they have with a vibrator is different from the kind they can give themselves with their hand, which is different from the kind they get from oral sex, and so on. Vibrators can be used as an alternative to, not a substitute for, flesh-on-flesh contact. If you feel anxious about falling too far in love with your vibrator, make sure to alternate using your digits (and his) with using the vibe.

Remember too that you're going to have to log a lot of vibrator hours to get you so used to it that nothing else will measure up. Even the most avid lifelong vibe users find they can still make themselves come without one. After frequent use, if you find that you have difficulty coming without a vibrator, or if you feel you've become hooked, give yourself a vacation from the vibrator for a little while, and go back to it when you are ready. That same rule applies if you've used your vibrator a lot in a short period of time and feel like you've "ruined" your clit. Repeated or prolonged use of a vibe can certainly leave your clitoris feeling raw, sore, overworked, or extremely sensitive. It may also leave it feeling desensitized or even numb. Don't be alarmed—normal feeling will return and you haven't done permanent damage. You've just worn your body out! Lay off the buzz for a while, give your clit a rest, and then take it easy, okay?

Men and Vibrators

Vibrators are not just for women—men too can enjoy their powerful, stimulating possibilities. Guys, you can use any of her vibrators to stimulate your balls, your perineum, and the base and shaft of your penis. If your partner uses a vibrator, you may want to try it out one day, alone or with her. Start with a low speed, and see how it feels buzzing against different parts of your genitals. There is also a great attachment for coil vibrators made especially for men called the "come cup." It looks like a rubber tulip and fits on the head of the vibrator. Lubricate the head of your penis and the inside of the cup. Stick the head inside the come cup and feel it vibrate against you.

Made of rubber or vinyl, vibrating sleeves are sheaths that vibrate around the penis. Lubricate your cock and the inside of the sleeve. Slip inside the sleeve and turn on the vibration, adjusting the level according to what feels good. Slide the sleeve up and down your shaft; the surrounding vibration adds an extra level of stimulation to any hand job.

Penis Pumps

For years, the penis pump has been one of the most popular sex toys for boys. They are available in several different styles. The simplest, most inexpensive kind is an all-in-one unit: a plastic cylinder and a tube leading to a pumping mechanism. Some of them also contain vibrating eggs for extra sensation. If you want to spend more money for more suction, there is a two-piece mechanism of a handheld hose pump and a detachable plastic cylinder (which is available in several different sizes). Here's how a penis pump works: the bottom of the cylinder creates a vacuum seal around the base of the dick, and with each squeeze of the pump, suction and pressure increases, and blood rushes to your penis. Slip your lubricated cock into its cylinder, and the suction gives you an erection and helps you maintain it. The advantage of a detachable cylinder is that you can pump up, then detach the pump, leaving the pressurized cylinder on. Some men like to use pumps to masturbate, but you might also consider trying it with your partner. Give her the controls, and she can be the one to pump you up.

Cock Rings

Made of a variety of materials, cock rings fit snugly around the base of the penis and the scrotum. Cock rings restrict the flow of blood out of the penis, a sensation that can be very pleasurable to some men. This restriction can give a man a firmer erection and help him maintain an erection longer than usual. Cock rings are an acquired taste. Some guys say that cock rings are uncomfortable and cut off their circulation, a decidedly unpleasant feeling. Cock rings definitely take some getting used to because they are indeed very tight.

Latex and metal cock rings are simple in design—they're solid, continuous rings that come in several different diameter sizes. You need to put this type of cock ring on *before* you get an erection. Once it's on and you get an erection, it's on for good. If you want to take it off, you've got a few options: let your erection go down; have an orgasm that will make your erection go down (this may be difficult if you are really uncomfortable); or cut the ring off with scissors (impossible for the metal variety without power tools—ouch!). There are also stretchy rubber rings which have a textured nub or several nubs on them; these are good for partner sex. Wear the nub on top of your cock and it will stimulate a woman's clitoris during vaginal penetration. These also need to be put on before you're erect.

If you are a newcomer to the world of cock rings, you may want to choose one that's easier to put on and take off. Leather, vinyl, and nylon cock rings have snaps or Velcro, so they are easy to adjust and remove. You should still put one on before you get an erection. The difference with this style is that you can adjust the size if it isn't comfortable or take it off altogether if you don't like it. But remember, like anything else that's new, the feeling takes some getting used to. Give it a fair chance before you throw in the towel.

There are also cock rings—made of hard plastic, rubber, or latex—that have a small bullet vibrator and a battery pack attached (which also serves as the controls). You can position the vibrator portion in two different ways. If you're masturbating, try it underneath the shaft for stimulation of the scrotum. With a partner, move the bullet on top to hit her clitoris during vaginal penetration. Keep in mind that some women may find this toy more frustrating than pleasurable, since rhythmic thrusting during penetration means the vibrator stimulates her clit on and off. To rectify the situation, try staying inside her and moving only slightly to achieve better contact between the vibrating portion of the cock ring and her sensitive clitoris. When you simply must start pumping again, she can switch to using her hand.

Experiment with different kinds of cock rings to see which ones work best for you and are the most comfortable to wear. In general, beginners should not leave a cock ring on for more than fifteen minutes to a half hour at a time. Like anything else, slowly work your way up to wearing it for longer periods of time.

Advanced cock-ring connoisseurs can look for a variety of styles that venture beyond the simple ring design—explore decorative studs, stimulating nubs, complex ball separators, and other fancy features.

Dildorama

Dildos are inanimate objects used for penetration. Many women find that they like to masturbate with dildos or use them in partner sex. The stereotype that men won't get a dildo for their wives because "then she won't need me anymore" is silly. Using dildos and other sex toys with a partner is a great way for men to increase their artillery. You can use a dildo to warm her pussy up for your cock. Or, for plenty of couples, their bodies are not always a perfect fit. Let's face it, as women get older, and especially if they have kids, everything gets bigger. Men already have anxieties about size, and when the vagina they are trying to please gets bigger, they can really freak out. Ladies, instead of dishing out cash for the misogynist cosmetic surgery that tightens your vagina to virginlike quality, simply encourage your sweetie to put something bigger than biology inside you. Or maybe you've got a different problem. Your man is very well endowed, and you're more than happy to comfortably accommodate him with your vagina; yet, when it comes to your ass, he's too large for it to work for you. Here's where a dildo that's smaller than him can mean you can still get the back-door attention you crave.

Men: If you come first and she hasn't yet, or she wants to come again before you're ready for round two, slip her favorite dildo inside her; it's a sure way to keep up with your multiorgasmic lover without taking Viagra. Or perhaps she'd like to experience double penetration without inviting a neighbor over. One cock plus one dildo can equal two happy holes for her (and for you).

Guys, don't think of a dildo as a cop-out. Expand your world and realize that sex does not always have to revolve around your penis. A dildo may not be part of your body, but when it's on the end of your hand, you're still the one who's going to get the credit for showing your girl a great time. And, take it from me, she will have a great time.

Selecting a Dildo

It used to be that there were few appealing dildos on the market; designed to look like realistic cocks, they were poorly made and, if they were trying to represent "the real thing," they weren't doing a very good job. But that was before women got their manufacturing hands on them! Today there are a wide variety of dildos for sale, and there is a small niche of women-owned and run companies making dildos that not only look and feel good, but get the job done right. From dirt cheap to top-of-the-line, dildos come in a variety of shapes, sizes, colors, textures, and materials. This potpourri makes choosing one difficult.

Your first consideration should be what the dildo is made of. The two most common materials are rubber and silicone. The biggest plus about rubber is economic: rubber cocks are pretty inexpensive. So, if you are dipping your toes into the dildo pool and aren't quite sure what you want yet, you can purchase a rubber dick for twenty dollars or less. If you're not satisfied or decide your eyes were bigger than your orifices, you can always buy another one. Most rubber cocks come in several colors, and vary from smooth or textured firm latex rubber to a clear, softer, jellylike rubber. The jellies look nice and the texture is super-soft and flexible, but eventually the surface tends to get small cuts in it. Jelly rubber toys are not long-lasting and will eventually need to be replaced. Because rubber dildos are porous and bacteria can linger on them, you cannot completely disinfect them; if you plan to share one with someone else, you should use a condom on it. Or you need to designate a toy as yours alone, and get another one for your lover. When you want to clean a rubber dildo, wash it in hot water and antibacterial soap or a sex-toy cleaner (sold most places where you can buy sex toys, these cleaners usually contain Nonoxynol-9). Let it air dry and remember that just because it's clean doesn't mean you should share it.

Silicone dildos are more expensive than rubber ones ($35–$100), but many people, me included, say they are worth the price. Silicone is an extremely resilient material and could last you an entire lifetime (some manufacturers even offer a lifetime guarantee!). Silicone dildos vary in their consistency, depending on the manufacturer, and can be soft, semifirm, or super-firm. There's also another edge that silicone has over plain old rubber: it conducts body heat and vibration. As you use the toy, it warms up inside you, and if you touch a vibrator to the end of a silicone dildo, you can feel the vibration all the way from the base to the tip. Silicone dildos come in a rainbow of colors (including metallics, glitters, and even ice-cream swirled designs!) and can achieve unique textures (like subtle bumps and ridges) that you cannot find in a rubber cock.

Companies like women-owned Vixen Creations make high-quality, top-of-the-line silicone toys in a wide variety of styles and sizes. The best thing about them is that they really work—you can tell they were designed and tested with sex in mind. All Vixen products come with a lifetime guarantee; if anything happens to it, you can return it for a replacement!

Silicone is completely nonporous, so it's very easy to clean and disinfect, which means that you can share silicone toys with different partners safely. To clean a silicone dildo, simply wash it in hot water and antibacterial soap, let it air dry, and it's good to go! You can boil silicone dildos in hot water for about three minutes, put them in the top rack of the dishwasher, or use a sex-toy cleaner with Nonoxynol-9. One other important tip to keep your silicone sex toys happy and healthy: do not use a silicone lubricant with a silicone toy without covering it with a condom—some silicone lubes have been known to ruin some silicone toys, and you don't want to take any chances!

The newest sex-toy material on the market is thermal plastic which folks may recognize from the brand name Cyberskin. These dildos have an extremely lifelike look and feel and they warm to body temperature; some say it's the closest thing to skin-on-skin sensation they've ever felt. The one drawback is in the difficulty of cleaning and maintaining these wonders. You have to wash the toy with hot water and antibacterial soap immediately after you use it (you do not want to leave it lying around overnight, trust me), then lightly powder it with cornstarch (*not* talc or baby powder) to return it to its original texture. Without the corn starch, the dildo becomes super-sticky, picks up all kinds of dust and lint, and is ruined pretty quickly. Some might call these high maintenance, but others say they are well worth it. Some women have also found that they have a bad reaction to this material, which may cause irritation and discomfort in the vagina. I'd suggest using a latex condom if you're sensitive to this material, but the condom sort of defeats the purpose of the super-realistic skin feel.

For those of you looking for a dildo that's beyond firm to downright rock hard, there are dildos made of clear acrylic, glass, wood, ceramic, and even metal. These rare beauties tend to look as good as they feel, but are definitely going to cost you. Each material is different, and you should ask the manufacturer or retailer about its unique features and cleaning instructions. Although there are several glass dildo manufacturers that I've seen, I can only recommend those dildos made of Pyrex-strength glass, which is safest and least likely to break (ouch!).

A company called Innerspace makes some of the most beautiful, artistic, and unique sex toys I have ever seen. These toys are handmade of crystal-clear, seamless acrylic, making them both stunning and functional. Acrylic (such as Lucite) is completely inert and very easy to clean. Once inserted into the vagina or the rectum, several of the dildos and the butt plug act as magnifying glasses, and with some light you can see everything. Perfect for art lovers and science geeks. Because they are super-firm and many models are curved, some women think they are ideal for G-spot stimulation and female ejaculation.

Once you've decided on your material, you need to think about how you want your dildo to look. If you want one that totally resembles the male member, you're more likely to find it in rubber or Cyberskin with balls, head, veins, and all. Mainstream companies like Doc Johnson, California Exotics, and Ben Wa specialize in rubber realistics. If you want realism, but will do without details like veins, you can find realistic silicone dildos as well.

Perhaps you're down with the phallic shape, but don't need it to actually look like a cock to work for you. There are plenty of dildos (made of rubber or silicone) that adopt that oh-so-traditional shape, but leave off any other references to its penile brother. They're usually available in bright colors, from the size of a large finger to a thick rod that's seven inches long and more than two inches in diameter.

Maybe you want to get away from the penis-substitute concept altogether, and have a dildo that looks (almost) nothing like a dick. Well, you can do that too. There are dildos fashioned into the shape of goddesses, cats, dogs, dolphins, and even shoes made by a company called Dils for Does that is known for its innovative designs in sex toys.

Another factor to keep in mind when choosing a dildo is the firmness; do you want soft, medium, or very hard? Remember that, depending on the manufacturer, the firmness of silicone can vary widely. Keep in mind that the firmer the dildo, the less flexible it will be. Dildos that are curved are designed to hit the G-spot in women and the prostate gland in men. If you want to wear a dildo in a harness, make sure it has a wide base and is compatible with the harness. (Look for details on dildo/harness sex in chapter 5 and sex-toy manufacturers in the Resource Guide.)

Using a Dildo

Women: As with any other sex toy, you may want to use a dildo by yourself first and figure out what you like. It's a great way to spice up your masturbation routine. Many women like to have something inside their vagina or ass while stimulating their clitoris, and using a dildo is often easier than using your own hand. Dildos can also be tools for learning during your self-loving sessions: if you had control over your partner's penis, how would you have it penetrate and please you? Experiment with different positions to see how they change the angle, depth, and sensation of the penetration.

If you've never used a dildo before, I'd start with a soft, flexible one. If you find it's not hard enough for your taste, you can always upgrade later. Use plenty of lube on the dildo—remember, it is a dry, inanimate object that will feel much better inside you when it's slick and rarin' to go!

Start slow and tease with the dildo; rub it on the outside of the vaginal opening, against the labia and clitoris. Start penetration with a well-lubed finger or two to get your body warmed up and ready for something bigger. Along with the dildo, you may want to add clitoral stimulation. Clitoral stimulation will feel great and help your vagina to relax and get ready for the dildo. Never just shove a dildo inside; there will be plenty of time for fast and furious later on, but in the beginning it's best to be slow, methodical, and gentle. If the dildo is curved, make sure the curve is going toward the navel, so you're hitting the G-spot.

You can choose to keep dildo play all to yourself, or you can introduce it into sex with your partner. As part of foreplay, he can tease you with a dildo. Men, don't assume it's only good for penetration. Rub it against her lips, her opening, and her clit. You can give her a hand job with a dildo, too. If your girl likes penetration to build from fingers to your cock, you can pick a dildo that's smaller than you that will relax and expand her pussy, get her aroused, and make the transition to your cock smooth and comfortable. While the dildo is inside her, you can go down on her, rub her clit with your fingers, or use a vibrator on her.

Women: if your partner has a sizable penis, starting out with a dildo can be a good way to warm up for it. If you have exhibitionist tendencies, use the dildo on yourself. Men, pay attention! By watching her closely, you could learn something about what turns her on and how she likes to be fucked. If she really likes her G-spot stimulation, but your fingers aren't enough to fill her and you can't seem to hit the spot with your cock, a curved dildo is the way to go. (See chapter 5 for more on G-spot stimulation.)

If you came, and she didn't, you could bring her to orgasm with clitoral stimulation. But, if she wants something inside her still, lube up a dildo, slide it inside her, and continue pumping away. It's like picking up where you left off. You can even get her into some wild positions that might not have been possible when the cock was attached to your body. Maybe you both came, but she's ready for round two before you are "up" to the task. A dildo is your knight in shining armor: give her eight orgasms in one night without having a heart attack.

Using Sex Toys Together

If you sense that your partner is not welcoming sex toys into your erotic life with open arms, don't be discouraged. You don't want to pressure anyone into doing something he or she does not want to do, but an open, honest discussion is appropriate and necessary to see if you can compromise at all. Ask your partner why he or she isn't interested in exploring this new realm of sexuality. Does she think it's weird? Does he believe that you'll fall in love with your vibrator and not need him anymore? Is she wary of changing your sex life in any way? Does he feel threatened that he isn't enough on his own for you? These are all common apprehensions that can usually be quelled with a little love and reassurance.

Approach a hesitant partner with compassion and respect, and explain that you want to try a sex toy to enhance your sex life. Assure your lover that your idea does not mean you think what you already have needs improving; instead, you simply want to experiment with something new. Sex toys are healthy, positive additions to anyone's sex life. If you and your partner are committed to each other and a growing sexual relationship, then you should be able to try almost anything at least once just to see what it's like.

Q&A

After I have a long night of vigorous sex or after several days of fucking, I seem to always get some kind of vaginal infection, either a yeast infection, a urinary tract infection (UTI), or both at once. It's becoming a chronic problem; what's wrong with me? Is there anything I can do?

Many different things cause yeast infections, including stress; antibiotics; tight panty hose, jeans, or underwear; pregnancy; menopause; even a high-sugar diet. Likewise, poor diet, birth-control pills, wiping back to front, pregnancy, menopause, stress, or a sudden increase in sexual activity can all cause urinary tract infections. If you are diagnosed with a yeast infection or a UTI, you need to make sure that you use all the recommended medication and you refrain from sex during the treatment. Women often feel better in a few days, but if they stop treatment or resume sex before they are fully healed, they end up aggravating the infection or becoming reinfected, and it's a vicious cycle. There are traditional medical treatments as well as homeopathic ones; whichever you choose, complete the treatment. Oil-based lubricants can lead to vaginal infections, so you should definitely use only a water-based lubricant, and I highly recommend you switch to one without glycerin, which many women are sensitive or allergic to. After a romp, I suggest you do two things: pee and wash up. Peeing will flush out any bacteria which may have gotten trapped in the urethra (which can easily happen, especially in certain positions or with deep thrusting) and can cause a UTI. Taking a brief warm soapy shower to wash your genitals will ensure that most of the lubricant is flushed out of your body, which means less of a chance of getting an overgrowth of yeast. I know it's not the most romantic thing in the world to do immediately after sex, but approach it this way: either encourage your lover to join you in the shower or remind him that a quick shower means you can remain infection-free.

HIT THE SPOT

G-Spot Stimulation and Female Ejaculation

What's the G for?

Before it was officially named by the scientific community, the G-spot was referred to in research and literature as a sensitive spot on the front wall of the vagina or as a spongy tissue surrounding the urethra. In a 1950 article, German gynecologist Ernest Gräfenberg became the first sex researcher to clearly identify this sensitive spot and its location. He was also the first to document female ejaculation, although he didn't call it that. When sex researchers Beverly Whipple and John D. Perry began publishing their research on the subject in scientific and medical journals, they decided to name the spot after Gräfenberg, and that is how it came to be known as the G-spot. Whipple and Perry put the G-spot on the map, so to speak, and their book with Alice Ladas, *The G Spot*, brought the spot and female ejaculation into popular consciousness.

The G-Spot

A woman's urethra is about 1½ to 2 inches long and is surrounded by spongy erectile tissue that contains paraurethral glands and ducts. (See illustration 6.)

The spongy tissue makes up the urethral sponge, also known as the G-spot. Let's clear up any misconceptions right away: every woman has a G-spot. The only thing that may vary is the size and location of the "spot," and how sensitive it is. Because it develops from the same embryologic tissue as the male prostate gland and produces fluid similar to prostatic fluid, the G-spot is often thought of as the female prostate.

Finding the G-Spot

The G-spot is located behind the pubic bone, around the urethra, and can be felt through the front wall of the vagina, about two inches inside the vaginal opening. The size of the spot varies—Perry and Whipple say from a dime to a half-dollar.[8] Opinions differ about the actual size of the G-spot, because, like the clitoris, the G-spot is connected to a network of nerves and tissue, so it's sometimes hard to say where it begins and where it ends. What we do know is that many women find a spot a few inches inside the vagina on the front wall to be very sensitive to stimulation and pressure. One thing to keep in mind as you begin the journey to find your own G-spot or your lover's is that the G-spot tends to swell when a woman is aroused. As it swells, it becomes a firm area that should be easy to distinguish from the rest of the vaginal wall. Swelling can take place very quickly or more slowly, depending on the woman. It is much easier to locate the G-spot once a woman is turned on. You might think the G-spot is "missing" if you look for it when its owner isn't aroused.

How will you know when you've found it? Many people

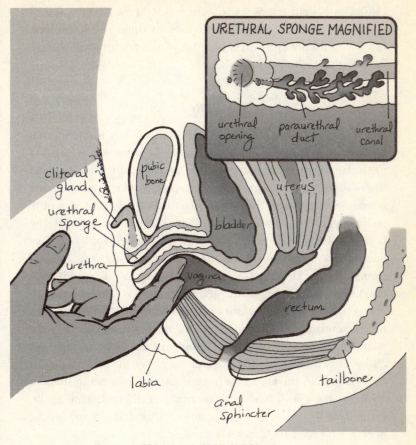

FIG. 6   G-SPOT ANATOMY

who've had the honor to touch a G-spot or two say that it feels spongy and slightly more textured (many people describe it as ridged) than the smoother-tissued area around it. When it is swollen, it protrudes slightly. Remember that the G-spot is not *on* the front wall of the vagina, rather it can be felt *through* the wall. Because you are feeling it through the vaginal wall, you need to apply a significant amount of deliberate pressure. A light touch just won't do much for the G-spot. If it's someone else's G-spot you're looking for, one way to know if you've found it is by the reaction of your partner. Many times when you look for it, you'll know you hit it because you're partner will squeal, "Yes! Right there!"

Having Your G-Spot Stimulated

When their G-spots are stimulated, many, if not most, women feel the urge to pee. That makes sense because you're putting pressure on the sponge around the urethra, which connects to the bladder. For some women, the urge to pee is an arousing sensation; they know they are not actually going to pee, so the feeling registers pleasure (rather than stress and anxiety) in the brain. Some women actually feel slightly turned on when they have to pee. Personally, I feel pressure around my urethra (as if someone's working my G-spot) when I have to piss, and it feels good. But when the entire genital region is engorged, with blood rushing to all the right areas, pressure on the urethra may be an entirely different sensation than when you're in a nonaroused state. Instead of feeling just the urge to pee, the entire area is electric with nerve endings, sensitive and alive. In other words, in this state, the pee feeling isn't like being stuck in a car in traffic and having to go really, really bad. That sucks. Instead, you're more aware of your entire genital region and the pressure on your urethra feels good.

A woman's response to G-spot stimulation (and any other erotic stimulation, for that matter) can also change. There are some times when G-spot pressure feels great, orgasmic, out of this world, and other times when the "spot" feels overly sensitive, too delicate for pressure, or it just doesn't feel good. In some cases, if you're not fully aroused to the point where the sponge has swelled, the sensation can change from pleasurable to just annoying. This strikes me as similar to stimulation of the clitoral glans (which makes sense since both are made of erectile tissue): if the clitoris hasn't become completely engorged with blood and swollen, and has retreated behind the hood, some-times direct stimulation—which normally feels great—feels too overwhelming. So, if your first experience with G-spot stimula-tion doesn't float your boat, you may want to try it again.

Keep in mind that you can dislike the "I'm gonna pee my pants" feeling but still enjoy G-spot stimulation. You just need to reassure yourself that you are not actually going to urinate, and surrender to the sensations. For some women, a full bladder or any pressure near the urethra is uncomfortable and irritating. For them, pressure on the G-spot often feels too sensitive, too unpleasant, and these women do not enjoy G-spot stimulation.

G-Spot Tools & Techniques

When it comes to G-spot stimulation, you have a number of options in the tool department. Fingers have an excellent advantage for this particular activity. For one, they are the best at being able to find the spot, since our sense of touch is keen and connected right back to the ol' brain. Fingers are diligent and talented little explorers, and I recommend that beginners always start with them. When using these little gems, remember that light touch doesn't work when it comes to the G-spot, you need to be direct and consistent with the pressure you apply to the G-spot. One of the best techniques to use with the fingers is the "come here" approach. With your fingers inside your part-ner and against the wall of the vagina, make a "come here" motion (toward you) with your fingers, almost like you are try-ing to pull the spot out of her. Some people also like to "dig" at the spot, but you better make sure your nails are well manicured or covered with a latex glove so you don't do any actual damage. Experiment with how much pressure, penetration, and move-ment she likes—ask her which techniques feel the best to her.

If you and your partner practice fisting (penetration with the whole hand), chances are some part of your hand will find the G-spot even if you aren't looking for it because her vagina will be so full. With your hand inside her, palm up with fingers curled down, you can use all four fingers to pull and stimulate the G-spot. Another technique I recommend for all you fisters out there is to turn your hand so that your thumb faces up and your fingers are curled to the left (this applies to right-handed people, reverse it for left-handers). Then, if you simply move your fist in and out of her, the knuckles of your thumb will press against the G-spot. (For more information about fisting, read the Q&A at the end of this chapter.)

Since the sex-toy industry has gotten much more savvy about women's pleasure, there are a number of dildos and vibrators designed with the G-spot in mind. In contrast to the traditional straight-as-an-arrow phallic shape, look for a very pronounced curve on a dildo or vibrator. These toys may have G-spot in their names or you can ask a sex-toy store employee for a recommendation.

Some women prefer a toy that's rock hard, since the G-spot responds to firm pressure. The Crystal Wand is an acrylic dildo created and marketed especially for G-spot stimulation and female ejaculation. Its unique shape—a perfect "S"—takes the concept of curves to a whole new level. Many women have told me that they had trouble locating their G-spots until they discovered the Crystal Wand. The combination of a rigid material and exaggerated curve may do the trick for you.

With any G-spot toys, make sure you work your way up to them with finger penetration first, and use plenty of lube. In-and-out movement with firm pressure will wake up that G-spot and make her sing. You may also want to try pressing the toy against the spot and using a pulling motion. Remember that you don't have to insert the entire length of toys that are five or six inches long—the G-spot is just a few inches inside. A steady rhythm and strong pressure will feel good, and the more aroused a woman becomes, the better it should feel.

Unfortunately for all you guys, the penis has a slight disadvantage when it comes to being a G-spot ace. No, it's not impossible to stimulate the G-spot with your cock, it's just a little more difficult. The shape of each cock is unique, but most men were not born with the dramatic curve ideal for this type of stimulation. But fear not, here's some advice to make you all expert G-spotters. It's all about getting the right angle, and that angle may depend on you and your lover's particular bodies and how they line up with one another in different positions. First, remember that the G-spot is not all the way inside the vagina, but only a few inches in. Fully penetrating her pussy, which may feel wonderful for all parties concerned, is not the best way to achieve G-spot stimulation. Instead, try entering her less than all the way; how far inside will vary, depending on the size of her vagina and the length of your cock. With the head of your cock, aim for that spot on the front wall as you move in and out of her. You may want to guide your penis with your hand in the beginning for better control. She can also help by directing you once you're inside.

While we are so diligently focused on the G-spot, let us not forget about the clitoris! Some women prefer G-spot stimulation by itself, while others appreciate both at once. Because all the nerves and tissues are connected, they play off one other, helping the entire genital region become stimulated. Many women find that simultaneous external and internal stimulation is like hitting the spot from both sides.

Positions to Hit the Spot

Because of where the G-spot is located (behind the front wall of the vagina), body position and the angle of penetration are important factors. Doggie-style position or a variation of it, with the head down and butt in the air, puts the body at an ideal angle and makes the spot easily accessible to a partner's fingers, a toy, or a penis. If your partner is behind you, he should aim downward and use a pulling motion toward himself.

If you like being on your back, the spot might be a little

tougher to find. Gravity can work against you. Try putting your legs up and to your chest. Or put a pillow under your butt to get a better angle. For those of you limber wonders, go ahead, show off and put your legs to your shoulders. Getting on top can afford you control over the angle of penetration, and you can simply tilt your body or rock your hips to find the perfect position.

Can you find your own G-spot? Yes, but it's not as easy as you may think. You'll probably have to experiment with different masturbatory positions before you find the one that works best for you. Women I know who can reach their own G-spots like to lie on their stomachs, squat (not very easy on the knees), lie on their backs with a pillow underneath their ass, or try solo doggie-style. Some women can stand and move their hips back to better reach it. Don't be alarmed if you can't reach it; the angle really does make it difficult to self-stimulate. Try a curved vibrator or dildo, which will be easier to maneuver and angle than your own hand. Or ask your lover to go on a little G-spot expedition with you; when someone else lends a hand, I bet you'll find the treasure, and won't getting there be fun!

Make Her Squirt!

Female Ejaculation Comes Out (of the Closet)

Female ejaculation is not a new phenomenon. Women have been ejaculating for a very long time (and it was documented as early as the 1950s), but there has not been a widespread public awareness of it. Many women have been creating spurts and puddles during masturbation and sex, but the problem is that most squirters don't know what is happening. Some attribute the extra dampness to an excess of lubrication and don't give it a second thought. Sadly, others think that they have lost control of their bladders and peed during sex. Some ejaculators believe they have an incontinence problem and go to a doctor seeking information and help. Unfortunately, many doctors don't know about female ejaculation or don't believe it exists; some have even performed surgery on women for incontinence, instead of reassuring them that it's a perfectly normal occurrence that happens to plenty of other women.

When the book *The G Spot* was released in 1982, Ladas, Whipple, and Perry provided original research—call it proof if you want—about female ejaculation. Beverly Whipple even made a video of research subjects ejaculating. A decade later, the lesbian video company Fatale released *How to Female Ejaculate,* an instructional video that clearly explained—and illustrated—the phenomenon. Yet a great majority of the medical and scientific community still refused to believe it or support further research. As a result, women are still being told by doctors that they are peeing, not ejaculating, and some are going under the knife to "correct the problem."

In order for doctors and scientists of mainstream institutions to accept the occurrence of female ejaculation, many would have to rethink their entire concept of female anatomy and sexual response. Instead, they dismiss female ejaculation or ignore it altogether.

Women have suffered self-doubt and embarrassment or shame and criticism from themselves, lovers, and medical professionals for too long. It is important for them and their partners to have clear and useful information about female ejaculation. What we learned about female ejaculation in *The G Spot* has been enriched by books like *The Good Vibrations Guide: The G-Spot,* by Cathy Winks, and *The Clitoral Truth,* by Rebecca Chalker. These books help reassure women and replace misinformation and doubt with research and facts about what our bodies are capable of.

Maybe you have always suspected that the puddle underneath you had some explanation. Perhaps a lightbulb has gone off in your head reading this, and you realize now that you (or your partner) has ejaculated before. In either case, the following information will give you new insight into what you are already capable of. It will reassure you that your body and sexuality are not abnormal in any way, and it may give you a few tricks to make your ejaculating experiences even better. Because many women may have had negative experiences with lovers in the past, been misinformed by health-care professionals, or felt ashamed that something was wrong with them, they need time to process the new, correct information. If this sounds familiar, give yourself (or your partner) a chance to get over your insecurities and accept your unique female ability.

If you are already a female ejaculator (and proud of it), use the information to answer any lingering questions, expand on your own knowledge on the subject, and add a few techniques to your squirting artillery. Hopefully, you'll learn a thing or two and continue to celebrate your ejaculation skills.

If you have never ejaculated before, read the information with an open mind. If you enjoy G-spot stimulation, you may want to take it one step further to ejaculation. If everything in this chapter is new for you, take in all in, and give yourself time to figure out if it's something you'd like to try. Female ejaculation is fun, it feels good, and it is another incredible way that women experience pleasure.

What Is Female Ejaculation, and All About the Fluid

During vaginal penetration when the G-spot is stimulated, the tissue of the urethral sponge fills with blood, becomes engorged, and swells. The paraurethral glands surrounding the sponge also swell as they fill with fluid. When a woman is very aroused and firm pressure is applied to her urethral sponge, the glands release the fluid through the urethra, and the woman ejaculates.

Studies have shown that there are significant differences in the chemical makeup of ejaculatory fluid and urine. Some researchers believe that ejaculate is made of prostatic fluid (similar to fluid produced by the male prostate gland) produced by the urethral glands; others think it is a chemically altered form of urine. Ejaculatory fluid is thin and liquidy and most often clear, colorless, or milky. It's usually odorless or may have a slightly sweet smell, and may taste sugary. The taste of women's ejaculate, as with all her vaginal secretions, depends greatly on her diet. The way most people know that ejaculate is not urine is by doing their own tests on the spot: feel it, taste it, or sniff the sheets, and you'll be able to tell right away. If you don't want to take my word for it, there is also some scientific proof as well.[9] It's difficult to definitively characterize ejaculatory fluid since there is so little research on the subject, yet from all of the research done, we know that it has different properties and a different chemical makeup than urine.[10]

So, if every woman has a G-spot, then why doesn't every woman ejaculate? Maybe the fluid is being released and women just don't know it. Here's one possible scenario: the sponge may be releasing ejaculate, but the amount is so small, it doesn't seem significant. Or women may attribute the wetness to any number of things—vaginal lubrication, secretions from the cervix, and that handful of personal lubricant she used—instead of ejaculatory fluid. Or the fluid could be a combination of all four substances. Some women feel the urge to pee right after sex. Another explanation is that as they pee, they may also be ejaculating right into the toilet bowel without knowing it.[11] Interestingly, Whipple and Perry suggested that women who ejaculate may be less prone to urinary tract infections or that women who hold back for fear of peeing and don't ejaculate can be more likely to develop a UTI.[12] Or maybe the fluid doesn't get released at all, and there has simply not been enough research to find out what happens to it or why some women do and some women just don't.

The chemical makeup is difficult to calculate. When a woman ejaculates, the fluid may combine with other substances, creating a combination fluid that is unique to each woman. All this pressure on the urethral sponge can also cause a woman to ejaculate *and* pee a small amount; if ejaculatory fluid is mixed with urine, obviously its properties change—it may be yellow in color or smell and taste more like urine. In some cases, vigorous G-spot stimulation can make her simply pee, without ejaculating at all. It's possible, but not likely.

Another reason that ejaculation is so hard to measure is that different women ejaculate in very different ways. In my bed, at sex parties and workshops, on adult movie sets, and in authentic videos, I have personally seen about fifty different women ejaculate. Many practiced and skilled ejaculators can actually shoot or squirt an impressive amount of fluid. I've seen women soak through towels and even gush like a low-pressure faucet. For other women, ejaculation is much less dramatic—the fluid seeps or leaks out of them, and they don't necessarily have a tremendous amount of control over it. These women may just find a small puddle under their butts after sex. Still others fall somewhere in between, delivering ejaculatory fluid in spurts or gushes, depending on the situation.

The quantity of fluid varies greatly depending on the woman. Some women may have bigger glands than others, or their glands may produce more fluid than others.[13] Whipple and Perry concluded from their research that the amount can range from a few drops to a quarter of a teaspoon.[14] I've witnessed women soak nearly half a mattress after they ejaculate several cups of fluid, while others release much smaller amounts of fluid. Some women are multiple ejaculators; they squirt once, then can be stimulated to squirt several times again. I can probably only fill a tablespoon with my own ejaculatory fluid. The important thing to remember is not to pressure yourself; however you do it is fabulous!

How to Make Her Ejaculate

Once you've located her G-spot, if you want to try to make her squirt, you need to apply direct, consistent, and pretty strong pressure to it. Remember, a gentle touch is not going to bring forth that precious fluid—you need to be pretty vigorous. If you are using your fingers, your hand should be facing palm up, fingers curved so you can create a pulling motion. Move those fingers back and forth, kneading and pulling at that spongy area. Keep it up until she tells you that she's ready to squirt. Sometimes, you can feel her start to bear down and then you know the dam's about to burst. Often, when a woman is about to ejaculate, you'll hear a particular sound as you work her G-spot. Instead of the traditional in-and-out music, this will be like a sloshing sound; it's unique, but difficult to describe. I want to say you'll know it when you hear it, but that's not any help, is it? Anyway, when she tells you or you feel her bear down or hear the sound, give the sponge one good pull, or you can try pushing up against it with strong pressure, and see what happens. If nothing happens, go back to what you were doing, give her more time to get revved up, and repeat all the steps as necessary.

If you are fisting her (have all five fingers or your entire hand inside her vagina), and you want to make her ejaculate, you need to change your hand position. Whether your palm is facing up with your fingers curled down or your hand is turned to the side with your thumb up, chances are you are taking up a whole lot of space in there. Often, with something as big as a fist (or an especially thick dildo, vibrator, or penis), you are most likely blocking the urethral opening, which means fluid can't come out. All you need to do is get out of its way. Slowly withdraw your hand from her vagina, then return with two or three fingers. Use your fingers to stimulate her G-spot, give it a few tugs, and watch her shoot her stuff. (For more on fisting, read the Q&A at the end of this chapter.)

You can also make her squirt with a vibrator or dildo. Again, choose one with a pronounced curve or an attachment made especially for G-spot stimulation. Make sure the curve is toward her navel and experiment with different positions until you get a good angle. Just putting it inside and pressing against her G-spot without moving it will not do the trick. Use the toy just as you'd use your fingers, with a firm pulling motion. She may also want to stimulate her clitoris while you are penetrating her.

Like I said before, hitting her G-spot with your penis is going to be challenging. I find it interesting that Whipple and Perry concluded that there was a higher rate of female ejaculation among women who have sex with women than heterosexual women.[15] They didn't expand on why this might be, but I have an idea: it's because lesbians who practice penetration are more likely to use their fingers, and finger fucking is a great route to female ejaculation. While straight men may dabble with their digits from time to time, they more often than not focus on their dicks, which, quite frankly, are not the best ejaculation tools for women.

Making her squirt with your cock may be difficult, but I know you're up for the challenge! On the set of an adult film, I saw porn star Kyle Stone employ a very interesting technique which I recommend you try. His partner in the film, actress (and known ejaculator) Jewel Valmont, was on her back on a table, and he was standing over her. He held his dick at the base and, with the bottom of his hand, curved it slightly upward toward her G-spot. He inserted only about half the length of his dick inside her so that the head of his penis would hit her G-spot. He used his dick almost like a dildo, controlling it and moving it very specifically and rhythmically with his own hand. After some spirited and consistent pumping, he pulled his dick out, and she shot ejaculate all over the place. So, lessons you can learn from Kyle: don't go all the way inside her. Remember, the G-spot is only a few inches in. Use your hand to control the angle and pressure of your penis. When she's ready to squirt, your penis may be blocking her urethra, so get out of the way and let her shoot!

How to Ejaculate

Women: in order to assuage any concerns or fears you may have about urinating, it's a good idea to pee before you have sex. A trip to the bathroom will reassure you that your bladder is fairly empty and you are much less likely to pee.

Some women ejaculate right away, others take more time to get there. When you are first starting out, take your time and be patient. Remember, once you are aroused and the sponge has swelled, it's much easier to find the G-spot. Some women who ejaculate find that it's easier to squirt once they've had an orgasm or two. For one thing, working your way up to an orgasm gets the juices flowing and gets the paraurethral glands producing fluid. Having an orgasm before you attempt to ejaculate will also help you to relax, which is absolutely necessary for you to do. If you are not multiorgasmic, then you may want to prolong foreplay, delay your orgasm, and get as worked up as possible.

As your partner stimulates your G-spot, take lots of deep breaths and relax. When you start to get the feeling like you are going to pee, tell yourself that you are not. Do not tense up or try to hold in your pee—this will make it extremely difficult to ejaculate. After plenty of G-spot stimulation, when you feel as if you might explode, many women say it helps to bear down, as if you are pushing something out of your vagina. Even if you still feel like you're going to pee, just let go. The worst thing that can happen is that you will in fact pee, but it's unlikely, especially if you just emptied your bladder before sex.

What does ejaculation feel like? Some women are very aware of exactly when they are ejaculating, and the moment it first begins. They feel like they have to pee, a sensation of pressure builds, they relax and bear down, and they release ejaculatory fluid. These women tend to have a well-developed PC muscle and good control over their ejaculation. Very experienced ejaculators as well as "gushers" (women who produce a large amount of fluid) usually fall into this category. Other women have less of a sense when ejaculation is happening.

When I first ejaculated, my girlfriend was working my G-spot with her fingers (she had a definite mission) and suddenly I got that feeling. It's a feeling I've had plenty of times during penetration and G-spot stimulation, a feeling like I was going to pee. I have always resisted the urge, held back, and many times even stopped the action to run to the bathroom. More often than not, I wind up on the toilet with a trickle or no pee at all. "I feel like I'm gonna pee," I said. "You're not going to pee," she reassured me. "Just let go." It was tough. I feel like I've been practicing for years to hold it in for fear I would pee on lovers who weren't exactly the golden showers type. But I had a profound amount of trust for her. So I did what she said, and I let go. Minutes later, I was coming. It felt like an altogether different kind of orgasm than I was used to. I had that climax feeling, but instead of being followed simply by a rush and pussy contractions, I felt this warm wave run through my insides. It just took over, and I went with it. When she took my hand and put it on the blanket underneath me, I was shocked. I made a puddle that soaked her beautiful bedspread!

The more you ejaculate, the more conscious you will become of what is happening, and when it happens. The more you relax and stay connected to your body, the better you'll be able to gauge where it's at and how the ejaculation process works for you.

If you'd like to try to ejaculate, one of the other things you need to do is make sure you are hydrated; as you can imagine, dehydration affects the production of all kinds of fluids in our bodies. Many women I know who ejaculate say that if they haven't had enough to drink or are dehydrated from exercise or something else, they definitely have a more difficult time ejaculating or they ejaculate much less fluid. So keep that tall glass of water or Gatorade by the bedside!

How to Make Yourself Ejaculate

You don't necessarily need a partner to ejaculate; many women can make themselves squirt during masturbation. Your ability to find your own G-spot and stimulate it enough to ejaculate depends on several factors: your particular body—the length of your arms, hands, and fingers; where your G-spot is located (since it does differ depending on the woman); how flexible you are; and your body position. If you'd like to make yourself come and squirt with your own hand, I recommend experimenting with different positions to see what works best for you. Follow the techniques I have already described, including firm pressure, the pulling motion, and bearing down. Some women find that it is much too difficult to reach their G-spot with their fingers. Others can find the spot, but cannot stimulate it vigorously enough to lead to ejaculation. I recommend using a dildo or vibrator with a pronounced curve or one that is specifically designed for G-spot stimulation, such as the Crystal Wand. Using a toy will take the pressure off, and you won't have to twist yourself into a pretzel in order to get at your G-spot!

Best Positions to Ejaculate

You should definitely experiment with different body positions for G-spot stimulation and female ejaculation, whether you are alone or with a partner. If you are going to lie on your back, it may help to put a pillow underneath your ass to get a better angle, and your partner should curve whatever he is penetrating you with upward (remember, we're aiming toward the navel). Doggie-style position or a modified version of it with your head down and your ass in the air is a good position for beginner ejaculators and their partners, since it provides a perfect angle for G-spot stimulation; your body is angled so that whatever goes into your vagina has a very likely shot at hitting the G-spot. When in this position, your partner should pull his fingers, his penis, or the sex toy back toward him.

Some women recommend the woman-on-top position for ejaculation because they can control the angle of their body, and the position of the spot in relation to their partner's penis; make sure to angle your body forward and lean into the penis, fingers, or whatever's inside you. Lots of women have great luck ejaculating while sitting, squatting, or standing up. Again, make sure to angle a finger, penis, or toy toward your navel, and you may want to move your pelvis or thrust your hips backward or forward, depending on which gives you better contact between your chosen tool and your G-spot. Don't expect greatness the first time around. Cut yourself some slack, it may take a few tries before you get the right combination of the perfect angle and levels of stimulation and relaxation in order to squirt.

Ejaculation Without G-Spot Stimulation

Thus far, my emphasis has been on direct G-spot stimulation, since that's how the majority of women ejaculate. From research (although far too little) and anecdotal evidence, we know that there are some women who can ejaculate without any direct G-spot stimulation whatsoever; they squirt from clitoral stimulation. So, how is that possible? Well, if you review your anatomy lesson and remember that the clitoris is much more far-reaching than just the clitoral glans, you realize that the G-spot is part of the clitoral system. Because these structures are close together and affect one another, stimulation of the glans certainly has an effect on the urethral sponge, and may cause it to fill with fluid.

Some of the same rules apply for ejaculation through clitoral stimulation: the more aroused a woman is, the more likely she is to ejaculate. Some women feel that if they press down right

Ejaculation Cleanup Tips

If you have experienced the wonder and amazement of a female ejaculator, you probably already know that it can be, well, very wet. And while wet is absolutely wonderful, washing your sheets every time you have sex is not. Thinking about cleanup beforehand makes things much easier—no one has to sleep in the wet spot (and trust me, that spot can be bigger and wetter than you imagine) and there's a lot less laundry for you to do. Here's a helpful guide to keeping it as dry as possible:

- *Light squirt:* a towel should do the trick

- *Medium-sized puddle:* disposable bed pads, aka "chucks," available in drug stores

- *Fountain of youth:* rubber sheets are the way to go

- *For the environmentally conscious:* try a washable absorbent pad

above the pubic bone, they can hit the G-spot "from the other side" and make themselves squirt that way. Many women say they can ejaculate after they've had an orgasm already by continuing to stimulate the clitoris.

Orgasm and Female Ejaculation

Ejaculating may feel like a big release, a genitally focused orgasm, or a deep full-body orgasm. Is ejaculating the same thing as having an orgasm? Well, like so many other sexual phenomena, that really depends upon the woman. When a woman ejaculates, her ejaculation may or may not be preceded, accompanied, or followed by an orgasm. Some women say that ejaculation feels like a release, yet it differs from how an orgasm feels; they may ejaculate first then later have an orgasm. Other women say that squirting is one kind of orgasm that they experience, different from other kinds of orgasms they have, but an orgasm nonetheless. For others, orgasm and ejaculation go hand in hand and seem to happen simultaneously. There are also women who experience orgasm, then continue to stimulate themselves to ejaculation. You do not need one for the other to happen—ejaculation and orgasm are not mutually exclusive.

Safer Sex and Ejaculatory Fluid

Since there is still much debate about the exact makeup of female ejaculatory fluid, some of you may be wondering what, if any, are the risks if you come into contact with it. Female ejaculate is another bodily fluid like vaginal secretions, semen, blood, urine, and feces. From what we know about it, female ejaculate does not have as high a concentration of HIV as semen or blood.[16] As you can imagine, there is no research on the risks associated with transmitting HIV, hepatitis, or STDs (like herpes, syphilis, gonorrhea, chlamydia, and others) through female ejaculate. If you are not fluid-bonded with your partner, you should protect yourself from ejaculate getting on any mucous membranes. That means using condoms, gloves, and barriers for oral sex.

Can Any Woman Ejaculate?

Whipple and Perry reported in the 1980s that as many as 40 percent of the women they surveyed ejaculated.[17] Let's compare ejaculation to another sexual phenomenon: the orgasm. Every woman has the necessary physical parts and capacity to have an orgasm. Yet some women have great difficulty achieving orgasm, or never do. Likewise, every woman has the necessary equipment to ejaculate, but not every woman ejaculates. Sometimes women may be too inhibited and afraid to pee to let themselves

Female Ejaculation on Video

Educational and Alternative

- *The Amazing G-Spot and Female Ejaculation*

- *Guide to G-Spot & Male Multiple Orgasm*

- *How to Female Ejaculate*

- *How to Find Your Goddess Spot*

- *The Incredible G-Spot*

- *Sluts and Goddesses*

- *Tantric Journey to Female Orgasm*

Mainstream Adult Stars Who Squirt

- Sarah-Jane Hamilton (*Squirt: The Cumming of Sarah Jane 1 & 2*)

- Alisha Klass (*Knocking at Heaven's Backdoor, Think Sphinc*)

- Taylor Hayes (*Taylor Hayes Anal All-Star 2*)

- Dasha, in various Vivid videos

- Several actresses in Greg Dark's *Psychosexuals*

ejaculate. Other times, they may ejaculate, but the amount of fluid is barely noticeable. I believe any woman can learn how to ejaculate. It's simply a matter of knowing more about your body and how it works, and practice, practice, practice. You may end up with the tiniest of puddles under your butt, and you may not become a shooting superstar. But you will learn about one more amazing thing women are capable of and you'll have plenty of fun trying to master this new trick. Don't pressure yourself to ejaculate because you think it's the cool new thing to do, it's the key to the best sex of your life, or you feel pressure from your lover. Do it because it feels good, do it because you want to, do it for you.

Q&A

What is vaginal fisting exactly? Can your whole hand really fit?

Vaginal fisting is the gradual process of putting an entire hand inside the vagina. Fisting gets a bad rap sometimes because its name is misleading: you don't start out with a clenched fist and push it inside a woman; instead, you begin with a single finger and work your way up. If your fingers are going walking, running, or dancing inside her vagina, make sure your nails are short and filed smooth. You want your hand to be as penetration-friendly as possible, and that means short nails with no sharp or rough edges. When you have your entire hand inside a woman, even the most minor hangnail can be felt on a grand scale, so I recommend well-fitting latex gloves to insure your hand is clean and smooth.

It is important for both partners to be relaxed for fisting to work. Tension can be felt intensely in your vagina and can make it impossible to have pleasurable penetration, especially on such a big scale. A warm bubble bath, a massage, and deep breathing are all good ways to relax—so is having sex and a few orgasms before you try for the fist! One of the best ways to get a fistee to open up to you is to get her so worked up she'll beg you to put the living-room couch inside. Warm her up with all your favorite tricks, the ones you know work like a charm—oral love, clitoral stimulation, vibrators, finger fucking, dildos, whatever. Remember to keep working her clit while you are working your way into her vagina. Deep breathing during fisting is also essential; many women take shallow breaths as they get turned on or even hold their breath for short periods. This may give you a temporary head rush, but it's just that—temporary. Breathing deeply will send blood rushing to all the right places, getting your clit nice and hard and your pussy open, ready, willing, and able.

When it comes to fisting, there is no such thing as too much lube. Thicker lubes tend to last a little longer, and the goopy consistency has a cushioning effect inside her vagina. As you work your way inside her, each time you add a finger, adjust positions, or just pause for a deep breath, add some more lube.

The fistee's body position must be both comfortable enough to endure for a long time (because it *is* going to take a long time) and afford you a good angle of penetration. Whether it is a sling suspended from the ceiling or pillows under her butt, experiment with different positions to see what works best for you. The fister can also experiment with different hand positions—palm up with fingers curled down, palm to one side, or fingers all together like a swan.

For those of you who may despise dialogue during sex, you're going to have to make an exception if you are going to put your entire hand in a girl. Talk to each other, find out what feels good and what doesn't, what's working and what's not. Experiment with positions, and most important, pay close attention to her body—it will tell you almost everything you need to know. Never force your way in; if you feel resistance, don't push the issue.

Everyone has to go at their own pace for fisting to be pleasurable (and to work!). Many people find that they can get all five fingers in, but then get stuck. The widest part of your hand is definitely the most difficult to get in. If you've gotten up to five fingers (palm facing clit), pour some lube in the palm of your hand and let it run right down to her opening. As you venture farther in, you'll find that your fingers will naturally curl down into your palm to make room for the rest of your hand. Fisting is always a gradual process, so don't rush it. Realize that sometimes it just won't work, and be ready for that. If you both breathe, go slow, practice a lot, and get her into a sexual frenzy, you might just be surprised what you can fit inside.

BACK-DOOR BETTIES AND
BEND-OVER BOYS

Anal Sex for Him and Her

Most of us have grown up with some negative ideas about our asses. For example, that your ass is a private part of the body that shouldn't be openly discussed or explored. Or that your ass is dirty and unsanitary. Many of us are taught that we shouldn't think about our asses in a sexual way, let alone enjoy them in a sexual way. There are also misconceptions about anal pleasure that run rampant in our culture. Only gay men have anal sex, and if straight men want it, then they are really gay. Or women have anal sex to please their male partners, but don't experience any pleasure of their own. Or anal sex is dangerous because it can cause physical damage to your body and is the simplest way to transmit disease. The truth is that the ass is one of the most overlooked erogenous zones in the body, and anal pleasure can be safe, healthy, and satisfying for men and women.

Myths and Facts About Anal Sex

Myth: It's messy and dirty.
Fact: If you're a healthy person with a normal diet, and you have a bowel movement before anal penetration, there will be only a trace amount of fecal matter in the rectum.

Myth: It means you're gay.
Fact: Plenty of people of all sexual orientations enjoy anal pleasure, and their desire for it does not change their choice in partners.

Myth: Women don't get off on it.
Fact: Women experience pleasure from the nerve endings in the anal area, indirect stimulation of the G-spot, and a combination of anal and clitoral stimulation.

Myth: It's dangerous.
Fact: If you do it right, you will not lose bowel control, develop hemorrhoids, or otherwise damage your ass.

Myth: That place is exit only.
Fact: Rich in nerve endings, the ass is a sensitive erogenous zone for men and women.

The Pleasures of Anal Sex

As discussed in chapter 1, anorectal anatomy is nearly identical in men and women, and the entire area—the anus, anal canal, and rectum—is extremely rich in nerve endings and sensitive to stimulation of all kinds, including penetration. Because of this level of sensitivity, exploring our asses can bring us incredible sexual pleasure. The one distinction in men and women's anal anatomy is that men have a prostate gland, which can be reached and stimulated through the rectum. Men experience pleasure from anal penetration through prostate stimulation as well as stimulation of the bulb of the penis and the perineum via the rectum. Although women don't have a prostate, they do have a G-spot. The G-spot is reached through the front wall of the vagina, but it can also be indirectly stimulated through anal penetration. Since all that separates the rectum and the vagina is a thin membrane, if you angle a finger, toy, or penis toward the front wall of the vagina, women still may experience G-spot stimulation.

In addition to the bundle of physical pleasure that anal stimulation brings, there are complex emotional and psychological issues that contribute to the erotic experience. For some people, the idea that anal sex is naughty, forbidden, and taboo is very exciting, and adds to their enjoyment of it. For others, the great amount of trust one must have in a partner heightens the physical pleasure; allowing your partner to penetrate you in this special place says, "Here is a delicate part of my body, and I trust you not to hurt me but to make me feel very good." That power exchange can be very intense for lovers. Anal sex is often represented in popular culture as violent and degrading; however, in reality, it can be extremely intimate, connecting, and spiritual.

Desire, Communication, and Relaxation

One of the most important ingredients for safe and pleasurable anal sex is desire. If you are not absolutely sure that you want your ass stimulated or penetrated, you cannot betray your body. Your ass never lies, and if you have any fears or misgivings, you will feel them on a physical level: your sphincter muscles will tighten and you won't be able to enjoy stimulation or have comfortable penetration. It's important to talk with your partner before the experience, so you can vocalize and resolve any issues or apprehension you may have. Once you clear the air, and agree that the receiving partner can stop any activities at any

Ten Ingredients for Great Anal Sex

1. *Desire:* For it to work, you've got to want it.
2. *Lube:* You cannot have enough of the slippery stuff.
3. *Relaxation:* Massage, meditate, breathe deeply, send your ass to an imaginary spa.
4. *Trust:* Talk to your partner.
5. *Arousal:* The more fired up you are, the more open your ass will be.
6. *Foreplay:* Don't forget to work all the other parts, too.
7. *Patience:* Don't rush, your ass has got all night.
8. *Pacing:* The slower you go in the beginning, the better it will feel in the end.
9. *Humor:* Smile, we're playing with our buttholes, after all.
10. *More Lube:* Go on, it will only make it better.

point, you'll both feel reassured and relaxed as you discover this newfound pleasure.

In addition to desire, communication is a critical part of pleasurable anal sex. No matter how well you know your partner, you cannot look into someone's eyes and understand exactly how she or he wants to be fucked in the ass. You need to ask, and your lover needs to tell you. A back-and-forth dialogue can really help both partners relax and not be anxious about what may happen next. The partner on the receiving end of anal penetration should absolutely be the one in control. You need to be the one to tell your partner what you want, and be specific: how slow or fast do you want the pace to be? Do you want penetration to be deep or not so deep? When you are ready to move on to more fingers, a bigger toy, his penis, or just something different, let your lover know.

Beyond communication, it does take a great deal of trust to have your ass penetrated. You are entrusting your partner with a very sensitive, delicate place in your body. If the penetrating partner does not know what he or she is doing, you can potentially be hurt. Anal sex can be very charged, intense, and emotional. That's why it's important for partners to be able to openly discuss their feelings, feel safe, and trust one another. The person receiving anal penetration can feel especially vulnerable, both physically and emotionally, and the partner giving anal pleasure must respect the receiver's wishes, needs, and limits. The penetrative partner may be afraid of hurting his or her lover. Again, communication and ground rules can help alleviate tension and reassure both people that it will be a safe and pleasurable experience.

Relaxation is critical to great anal sex. Living in a very stressful world, we hold stress in different places in our bodies, and the ass is one of the most popular places to keep stress in—that's where the expression "tight ass" comes from. Whatever it takes for you to relax—whether it's deep breathing, candles and incense, meditation, or visualization—letting go of tension in the body and putting the day's activities out of your mind will help you physically and mentally prepare for anal sex. Some people also like to have an orgasm before they begin exploring anal pleasure; it's another great way to get aroused, release tension, and relax the body.

Everyone must go at their own pace for anal sex to be pleasurable, and when both partners are patient, it's much easier for everyone to relax (especially the receptive partner). Anal sex is also a gradual process of exploration. We *progress* to anal penetration. Anal sex is not a choice activity for a night when one or both of you just want a quickie, or someone has somewhere to be. If you are anxious or stressed out about anal sex, sex in general, or the presentation you're giving tomorrow at work, it's probably not the best time to experience anal eroticism.

The Mess Factor

The number one question I am most often asked about anal sex is, "Won't it be messy?" Most people are anxious or reluctant to explore their partner's ass for fear that they will, well, step in shit. If you recall from the anatomy lesson in chapter 1, beyond the rectum is the colon, and you cannot reach the colon without something much longer than a penis or a dildo. The colon has no sexual function, but it is important to acknowledge how it relates to anal penetration. Feces are stored in the colon and move into the rectum when you're ready to have a bowel movement. The rectum is not a storage facility. This is the case for people with normal diets, good bowel habits, and no gastrointestinal problems. So, if you feel like you have to go to the bathroom, and you do, there will not be very much fecal matter in the rectum. On the other hand, if you feel like you have to go to the bathroom, but you do not and instead have your ass penetrated, well, there is likely to be a mess. The moral of this story is listen to your body and go to the bathroom when you feel the urge. It is a good idea to empty your bowels before you have anal sex.

Some people like to have an anal douche or enema before anal sex. Know that you do not have to have an enema in order to have relatively clean anal sex. Having a bowel movement and a warm soapy shower to clean the external area should do just fine. If you do want to have an enema, there are several different kinds. You can buy a Fleet enema or a plastic bulb syringe at the drugstore. If you use a Fleet, empty the plastic bottle first—it contains a liquid laxative you don't need to use—and refill it with plain warm water. Always follow the instructions on the box. If you are going to use an enema, you should have one at least three hours before you have anal sex. Do not overdo it on enemas. I don't want to see any of you at an Enema Addicts Anonymous meeting. Enemas rinse all the bacteria out of the bowels, the good, the bad, and the ugly (including some that's benefi-

Enema Tips

To give yourself an enema, you can use the Fleet or a bulb syringe. You may want to use an enema bag (a water bottle with a tube attached to it), which rinses farther up into the rectum. Fill the bag with plain warm water only; never use laxatives, wine, beer, coffee, or any other exotic enemas you may have heard about—they will make you sick. Giving yourself an enema this way takes a little more skill (and maybe even an assistant). In addition to your enema bag and tubing, you need a hook of some kind and a place to hang the bag that will be within easy reach of your butt and about eighteen to twenty-four inches above your ass. Find a position that's comfortable; you may want to try squatting, lying on your side with one leg pulled up to your chest, or kneeling with your ass up, head down. Use some water-based lubricant on the tip of the nozzle; this goes for the bulb syringe as well, and the Fleet enema's tip is pre-lubricated. Gently insert the tube into your ass.

With a Fleet or bulb syringe, simply squeeze the bottle or bulb and the water will flow into your rectum. With an enema bag, you need to release the gauge on the bag until water begins to flow at the desired pressure (very low pressure is best). Let yourself fill up until you feel like you've had enough. When you feel full, close the gauge and take the tube out. Wait a little while (the time varies depending on the person) until you feel like you need to have a bowel movement, then go to the toilet. Repeat the enema several times until only clear water comes out.

An enema loosens everything in your bowels, and often after you feel like you are completely cleaned out, you'll have an urge a little while later only to discover there was more in there. This is the second wave, and you don't want it to happen while you're in the throes of anal pleasure! Giving yourself an enema in the morning before a hot date that night is fine. If it's not disposable (like a Fleet) then clean your enema equipment well, and do not share it with a partner.

cial), as well as the thin layer of mucus that helps protect the delicate lining of the rectum. Enemas can wear your body out, so you don't want to have too many. An enema may feel strange or slightly uncomfortable, but it should never be painful. If you have cramps, the temperature of the water is probably too cold. If you have other pain, stop at once.

Preparation and Techniques

As you read in chapter 3, lubricant can greatly enhance all kinds of sexual experiences. When it comes to anal penetration, lube is not a luxury, it is an absolute necessity. Unlike the vagina, the rectum is not self-lubricating. If it feels lubricated to you, that's probably the mucus that lines the rectum and some sweat, but it's not enough to have pleasurable penetration. Spit will not do the trick either—you need a store-bought lubricant. There are dozens of kinds to choose from, and you can reread chapter 3 for all the details. I find that thick, water-based lubes that are the consistency of hair gel work the best for anal penetration. Lubes like ID, Wet, Maximus, Foreplay Lube DeLuxe Gel or Cream, Probe Thick and Rich, and Slippery Stuff Gel, among others, stay wet longer than their liquidy counterparts and also provide some cushioning for the delicate rectum. (There's no such thing as too much lube for anal play, and it may get a little messy. Moistened unscented baby wipes are a great way to clean up. They can also help prevent lube from the ass dripping into the vagina, which may cause an infection; one swipe of the wipe, and you're all clean!)

The tissue of the anal canal and rectum is quite delicate and much less resilient than the tissue of the vagina. The delicacy of the rectal tissue is a blessing and a curse: a blessing because it makes the area incredibly sensitive to all kinds of touch, but a curse because we do need to take extra care during penetration. Without proper warm-up and preparation, you can tear the lining of the rectum and cause irritation, discomfort, or pain. But with a few precautions, you can prevent any tearing or pain and focus on pleasure instead.

When done correctly, anal sex will not cause permanent damage to your rectum. As I say in my video: let's put this myth to rest once and for all. If you have a lot of anal sex, you are not going to end up in adult diapers. In others words, frequent backdoor banging—when done properly with care and lots of lube—will not lead to enlarged and/or loose sphincter muscles or a loss of bowel control. In fact, having a lot of anal sex may do just the opposite: you may find that you actually have *better* bowel control than you did before. You see, in order to take something inside your anal canal and rectum, you have to learn how to relax your sphincter muscles. The more you practice controlling these muscles, the more you are exercising and toning them (just like any other muscle). You are not stretching out or loosening the sphincter muscles, you are simply relaxing them to allow penetration.

Plenty of foreplay and warm-up go a long, long way toward achieving satisfying anal penetration. Getting your partner revved up in whatever ways really do the trick is half the battle; once someone is aroused, their genitals are engorged, their muscles are relaxed, and they are more receptive to penetration. Even if the goal of the evening is anal sex, you don't have to dive right in. Don't neglect other sweet spots on his or her body.

I recommend that you begin exploration of the ass with a tool that's small, gentle, and connected to a brain: your finger! I like to think of my finger as "my man on the inside." He's got his hard hat with the big light on top and is gonna tell me what's going on in there. To penetrate someone with a toy, it's a little like flying blind—you don't know what the person feels like on the inside, and you don't know how the body responds to what you're doing since the toy has no sensors. Your fingers, on the other hand, can give you a firm grasp of this new and mysterious territory, telling you where everything is (remember that all-important curve of the rectum), how the rectum feels, and what it responds to. In order to make sure your fingers are going to feel good rather than wreak havoc inside, you need to have a good manicure—clean, short, well-filed nails. If you aren't content with your nails, then slip into a latex glove. Gloves make your fingers smooth and protect the ass from rough edges, torn cuticles, and other potential dangers. Ladies, if you're going to let your fingers do the walking and you've got a lovely manicure of real or fake nails, don't despair. Put cotton balls into the tips of the fingers of a latex glove. You lose a little bit of sensitivity, but you can reassure yourself that you won't tear through a glove or irritate your partner's ass.

When you are ready to proceed, rather than insert your well-lubricated finger straight inside as if pointing to something, touch the pad of your fingertip to the anus. This feels soft and nonthreatening and will likely cause the anal opening and sphincter muscles to relax and allow something inside. Slide your finger inside only up to the first knuckle and just stay there, letting the butt get used to having something inside it. Remember that everything registers bigger and bolder than it really is when it is inside the butt, so never go too far too fast. Don't rush it.

The more time you are willing to devote to a gradual, gentle exploration, the more your ass will benefit in the end. It's all about working your way up. One of the reasons that I made my video, *The Ultimate Guide to Anal Sex for Women,* is that I believe people learn things from adult films. Too often in videos the man shoves his huge penis right into a woman's ass without lube or warm-up. The truth is that even the most experienced anal receivers and the professionals need to work up to a penis. The problem with most anal porn is that all the lube and warm-up with fingers and toys either happens off camera or ends up on the editor's cutting-room floor. No one can go from zero to sixty in five seconds; it's just not possible! Too many couples try to rush anal penetration, and it ends up being painful for the

What Happens If It Hurts?

1. There may be too much friction. Withdraw, add some more lube, and see if it feels better.
2. Stop the movement of fingers, cock, or toy, but stay inside; see if the pain subsides.
3. Decrease the number of fingers you have inside or use a smaller toy.
4. Withdraw and focus on more external stimulation—a hand job, oral sex, more foreplay.
5. If you need to, stop the activity altogether. Relax, take some deep breaths, listen to your body.

receptive partner. Of course, after the first negative try, no one really wants to experience it again.

Anal penetration does not have to hurt—not even a little. If it hurts, you aren't doing it right: either the person isn't warmed up or relaxed enough or you're not using enough lube. Pain is your body's way of telling you that whatever is happening isn't working. Honor and respect your body, and if you feel pain, stop what you are doing. There is a fine line between pain and discomfort, and everyone's line is different. Anal penetration may feel strange at first. Your ass is used to expelling things out of it, not taking objects into it. So when first-timers are penetrated, they sometimes feel as if they need to have a bowel movement. I suggest you go to the bathroom and see what happens. Most likely, you really don't have to go, because hopefully you had a bowel movement before sex. It's just your body attempting to reorient itself toward this new feeling. The more you experience anal penetration, the more this urge to "go" will subside.

Anal Sex Toys

In addition to fingers and penises, there are a variety of sex toys you can also use on your ass (see illustration 7).

Whatever kind of toy you select, it must have one important feature: a flared base. Perhaps you have heard rumors about people "losing" objects in their rectums and rushing to the emergency room. Or maybe you've seen one of several Web sites which document X-rays of different items people have put in their rectums. While part of this is pure urban legend, the truth is you *can* get something lost in your ass if you aren't careful. Once you are aroused, your pelvic muscles contract, and this could cause your ass to "suck" something all the way inside it. The best way to prevent your own trip to the ER is to use a toy with a flared base, since the base will prevent it from going beyond the rectum and into the colon.

As their name tells you, butt plugs are made expressly for anal pleasure. The traditional shape of a butt plug looks like a teardrop with a thicker bottom or a skinny pear shape. There are variations on the shape, including a lopsided diamond shape and a bulbous head with a long neck. Above the wide flared base, the plug's neck has the smallest circumference, designed to allow the sphincter muscles to close around it. Butt plugs may be smooth or textured with ridges, ripples, rings, or bumps. Butt plugs are usually made of latex rubber or silicone; there are also clear acrylic (similar to Lucite), glass, wood, ceramic, and even metal plugs, but they are for more experienced anal players. Butt plugs come in a whole bunch of sizes—remember that it is always best to start small and work your way up.

If you like the feeling of something just being in your ass, and appreciate the fullness and pressure without necessarily moving in and out, than you would probably love a butt plug. Butt plugs are meant to go in and stay in. Once you slowly slide a well-lubed

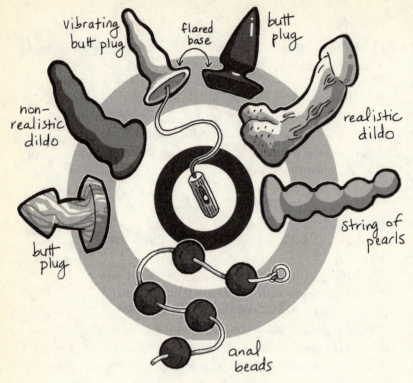

FIG. 7 ANAL SEX TOYS

plug inside the ass, you can then move on to something else—clitoral stimulation, a blow job, vaginal penetration, whatever you'd like—and the butt plug will continue to stimulate without a lot of work on your part.

If you have a butt plug in, you may find that when you get really aroused or during orgasm, the plug inadvertently slips (or even shoots!) right out of your ass. While this may be surprising or embarrassing, don't be alarmed, it's pretty common. Remember that during arousal, your genital muscles contract, and those contractions may actually push a plug out of your ass. This doesn't necessarily mean that the plug is too small and you need to run out and upgrade—it's just a signal that you are very turned on!

Butt plugs are also a great way to warm up the ass for bigger things to come. Putting in a plug and leaving it in for a while lets the ass get used to having something inside it. The ass opens up and relaxes around it, and when you take it out, you're ready to move on to something more.

That something more may be a dildo. As you read in chapter 3, dildos come in all shapes, sizes, colors, styles, and materials. If you like your anal penetration to include in-and-out-style fucking, then a dildo is the right tool for you. Any dildo with a flared base is appropriate for anal penetration. If the dildo is curved, make sure the curve is always going in the direction of the front of the receptive partner's body to insure stimulation of the prostate or the G-spot.

Some butt plugs and dildos are also vibrators. Vibration not only stimulates the genitals and feels really good, but it also relaxes the body. That's why so many vibrators are sold as massagers. Some people find that the added feature of vibration helps them to relax the sphincter muscles and makes anal penetration easier and more pleasurable.

There is one exception to the flared base rule: anal beads. Made of either hard plastic or rubber, there are usually about five beads (which can range from the size of marbles to the size of super balls) on a string with a large ring on the end of it. There are also even larger ones—I've seen them the size of tennis balls—but they are unrealistic and potentially unsafe; stick with a reasonable size. For some people, the moment when the sphincter muscles relax and let something inside the ass is the most arousing; with anal beads, you can experience that moment five times.

Lubricate the beads, and insert them slowly and gently, one at a time. Once the beads are in, you'll be able to feel them as you move on to manual stimulation, oral sex, or vaginal intercourse. Some people like to pull out the entire string of beads

Anal Sex Tricks

- *Round Two:* Have anal sex after she's had an orgasm. She'll be relaxed, and her body will be aroused.

- *Practice, Practice:* Add a butt plug to your masturbation routine to help your body get used to anal penetration.

- *Plug It In:* Use a vibrator to stimulate her anal opening and relax the area before penetration.

- *Spank Her:* If your gal likes to be spanked, before anal penetration is a great time to put her over your knee. Reddening her butt cheeks will send blood rushing right there and stimulate her ass.

- *Smooth, Please:* Use a regular condom, as a textured one might irritate the delicate lining of the rectum.

right before they orgasm—it sends them over the edge. Others pull them out during or immediately following orgasm. Just don't pull them too fast or you can tear that delicate tissue.

A few words of caution if you're interested in anal beads. Many anal beads are inexpensive and poorly made. The hard plastic kind may have sharp edges at the seam of the ball that can irritate or tear the tissue of the anal canal and rectum; some people also complain that the knots in the string feel uncomfortable. These type of beads are impossible to completely disinfect, so never share them with a partner; each person should have his or her own. If you love beads, but have concerns about the edges or cleaning them, there are a few solutions. Vixen Creations is the only toy manufacturer that makes an entire string of anal beads dipped in silicone. Silicone means they are a snap to clean, and the beads are super-smooth. Other companies have dildos that take off on the idea of anal beads, featuring several round rubber orbs linked with rubber—the same great feeling with no sharp edges or hard-to-clean string.

If the receptive partner is a woman, it's important that nothing go directly from her ass into her vagina; that's a great way to get a vaginal infection. Whether it's a finger, penis, or sex toy, if it has been in her ass, make sure you either wash it thoroughly with hot water and antibacterial soap or put a new latex glove or condom on it.

Positions for Anal Sex

In this section, I may focus a little more on men penetrating women in the ass, but these positions will work no matter who's pitching and who's catching. Guys, you are not off the hook. You get your chance to take it in just a few pages.

There aren't any secret positions for anal penetration that you probably don't already know about. In other words, any position you've been in for vaginal penetration is worth a try for anal penetration. Since everyone has individual needs, tastes, and desires, it is important to experiment with all kinds of positions to discover what works best for you and your partner. Different positions offer different features, from endurance and comfort to a certain angle of penetration or the feasibility of deep thrusting. When considering which may work best for you, think about how comfortable both partners will be in a position, and if both of you can stay where you are for a while. What is the best position for anal sex? I get asked that question almost everyday, and the answer is: the one that works best for you.

I am partial to the doggie-style position for beginners. This position, with the receptive partner on hands and knees—or slightly modified with head down and ass in the air—and the insertive partner behind offers some important pluses. For one, the penetrator can clearly see where he's headed, which is important especially when you are negotiating between two openings that are very close together. When the receptive partner's head is down, the body creates a perfect angle of penetration to hit the G-spot. In this position, you can reach around and rub her clit or she can do it herself.

Doing it doggie-style also does plenty for the more experienced, and gives both of you lots of pelvic movement for both partners. The receptive partner can move back on a penis from this angle. She can also be in control of the action if he does less of the movement, and lets the receiver come to him. He can do a lot of deep, hard, or fast thrusting, and doggie-style can be anything *but* a gentle first-time fuck.

Yet another variation on this position has the receptive partner on her stomach with either her knees bent or her legs straight. Although this one may seem awkward on first try, it just takes a little practice. This too is a good position for medium or deep penetration because the rectum is in an optimum position for pretty smooth entry (as long as you don't forget that important curve!).

Missionary position finds the receptive partner on her back and the insertive partner on top. Because both partners face each other, this makes it easier to communicate, especially non-verbally, plus you can attend to other parts of your partner's body—suck on her nipples, kiss her neck, rub her clit. Many people in the receptive position like missionary-style anal penetration because lying on their back is either more comfortable or allows them a sense of surrendering to their partner.

The receptive partner may find that a pillow under her butt makes for easier penetration, and she can bend her knees or bring her legs either to her chest or rest them on her partner's shoulders. Although the latter position may create a better angle for entry, it is often one that even the most flexible among us find hard to sustain. If your partner cannot provide clitoral stimulation, you can do it yourself with your hand or a vibrator.

If the receptive partner wants to control the angle and depth of penetration, then she should try being on top. Straddling the insertive partner, she can sit straight up, or lean forward or backward. Again, facing each other means you can talk as well as stroke, rub, pinch, and stimulate other parts of each other's bodies; this position is also great for clitoral stimulation. Receptive partners can really take the lead in this position and be in charge of the depth, the amount of movement, and the rhythm.

Insertive partners who are inexperienced, nervous about how to penetrate their partners anally, or fearful of hurting their partners may find this position most relaxing because the receiver can do much of the decision making and the work. The partners on the bottom often report liking this position best because they get a great view of their partner and can watch her as she receives pleasure.

Spooning is a position in which both partners are on their sides, either facing each other or the same direction. This position is comfortable, flexible, easy to maneuver, and it gives both partners good control over the angle and depth of penetration; it's an ideal position for partners who are of very different heights or sizes. Some people find that lying side by side gives them greater access to their partner's vagina, clitoris, penis, balls, and to all parts of each other's bodies for exploration and stimulation. You don't get the depth of penetration this way as with other positions; however, spooning is good for a long, slow anal fucking session, where no one's in a rush to get somewhere. But don't get me wrong, you can still have ecstatic orgasms this way, especially because you can be stimulating lots of other parts while you're doing your partner's ass.

These are a few of the most common positions, but by no means all the possible ones. There are plenty more for you to explore and try out. Some people like to reverse the receptive-partner-on-top position and face the same direction rather than each other. Couples who are similar in size may find they can do it standing up or with one person bent over a bed or table. Think of each new position as an opportunity to explore different depths, speeds, rhythms, and dynamics; there's lots of erotic territory you'll find simply by changing your point of view.

Traditional Butt Fucking

I want to stress that anal pleasure comes in many different forms, from licking and external stimulation, to penetration with fingers or toys. Anal sex should not be equated only with his cock in your ass. However, that said, if his cock in your ass is the desired goal, here are some tips to get you on the right track. (Pay attention, girls, you can change the pronouns and use many of these techniques on his ass, too.)

Start with plenty of foreplay—work her clit, lick her pussy, play with her breasts, and get her as excited as possible. The more turned on she is, the more engorged her genitals will be. When everything is wet and swollen, it's also relaxed and more receptive to penetration. Play with her butt cheeks—squeeze them, stroke them, maybe even spank them a little. Spread some lube on her anal opening and the perineum; stimulate the external area to get her focused on feeling pleasure in her ass. When you begin to penetrate her with one well-lubed finger, go deliciously slowly. Work her clit with your mouth or your finger or a vibrator while your finger is in her ass, or guide her hand between her legs for self-stimulation. Remember, clitoral stimulation will not only help relax her, it will also make anal penetration feel better. Some women tighten their sphincter muscles when their clits are being stimulated, having the reverse effect—she'll let you know if the stimulation is helping her open up or if she's clamping around your finger instead.

When you first get inside her, just past the sphincter muscles, just go up to the first knuckle and stay there. Let her ass get used to the feeling of your finger. One trick I like to use is where I gently press in what I call the "North-South-East-West" motion: up, down, and side to side with a subtle amount of movement and pressure. As you proceed farther inside, remember to angle toward the G-spot; you can even try rubbing the front wall of the rectum for more G-spot stimulation. Let her be the one to tell you when she wants more fingers. Slowly withdraw your finger, add more lube, then slide two fingers inside gently. Again, begin with the pad-of-the-finger trick, and let her get used to the sensation of more fingers in her ass.

Once she's more relaxed and used to the feeling, you can start to move in and out. Remember that the ass is more sensitive, so proceed more gently than you may be used to when finger-fucking her vagina. On the road toward putting your cock in her ass, you can proceed a few different ways:

- Continue with finger penetration, adding fingers two, three, and maybe four; or
- After two fingers, switch to a slim dildo which you move in and out of her ass; or
- Slide a well-lubricated butt plug slowly inside her ass. Once it is all the way in, play with it a little bit by tapping on the end of it or moving it slightly. Then, give her some clitoral stimulation or maybe vaginal penetration. Perhaps she can suck your dick or give you a hand job. After the butt plug has been in for a while, you can carefully slide it out. Her ass should be relaxed and ready for you.

After the warm-up period, lubricate your penis and re-lube her anus. Place your cock at her anal opening and hold it with your hand to help you guide it. Again, you have a few options:

- Have her move her body toward your cock (forward or backward depending on your positions), while you guide it inside.
- Rub your cock against her opening. This external stimulation should relax the anus. As the sphincter muscles contract, the opening appears to "wink" at you. As it winks open, take the opportunity to slide in.

- Press your cock against her opening and gently push against it (she may want to either relax or bear down in order to let you inside).
- Penetrate her ass with your finger, withdraw it, and while her anus is open, gently insert your penis.
- Have her stimulate her clit as you penetrate her. This will relax and arouse her, making penetration easier.
- Deep breathing will help her relax and concentrate on opening her ass to you as well as circulating blood to her genitals. (Taking shallow breaths tightens the muscles and inhibits the engorgement process.)
- Girls, if he's having trouble hitting his intended target (hey, those two holes are close together and it's slippery with all that lube), wrap your fingers around the head of his cock and help to guide him inside your ass.

When you first get inside her ass, don't go too deep. Again, you want to give her ass an opportunity to get used to your penis. Keep your movements slow, gentle, and subtle at first. When she's ready, you can venture farther inside and start some slow thrusting. She should tell you if she wants you to go deeper or faster or both. Then, it's simply a matter of exploring what feels good for both of you.

Anal Pleasure for Men

Let me admit my bias about male anal pleasure right off the bat. Guys: getting fucked in the ass is one of the greatest gifts you can give a woman and yourself. First, there is the purely physical prize that awaits you when you are on the receiving end of anal pleasure: incredibly arousing prostate stimulation. Too many men still have not experienced the wonders of their prostate gland. For many of you, your first foray into the land of anal penetration probably took place in a sterile white room, on a paper-covered table. Your proctologist squeezed a lump of K-Y onto his latex-clad hand and shoved his finger up your ass. It wasn't erotic, it didn't feel particularly good, and you weren't even attracted to the guy. All this happened five minutes after words like "prostate cancer" and "rectal exam" were uttered. Some turn-on. Now you know how women feel at the gynecologist's. Put this experience out of your mind—it was a medical exam. I'm talking about mind-blowing sex.

But in order to have this mind-blowing sex, most men must first get over a lot of shame and fear and embrace all the ass has to offer: those nerve endings, that sensitive tissue, and the pleasures of the prostate. Remember, a few inches inside the rectum and toward his navel, the "male G-spot" and a world of ecstasy awaits.

Since anal pleasure is still taboo in American culture, anyone who admits to being a backdoor betty is on the front lines of sexual liberation. As women, since we are already positioned as the receptive, penetrated partner, we need only reorient ourselves to focus on the *other* orifice. The man, on the other hand, is the penetrator, the active partner, the pencil to her sharpener. Anal sex is a unique opportunity for men to be penetrated—the other side of the fence for those of you usually dishing it out. Giving your body over to a woman in a (w)hole new way requires extreme trust; plus, men must also confront some of the baggage that comes with a desire for anal pleasure. Reassure yourself that wanting to be a bend-over boyfriend does not make you gay, kinky, or immoral. Some men may feel particularly submissive when a woman "does" them; however, you don't have to be passive to be penetrated. I encourage you to work through any issues you may have about your sexual or gender role, and come out of an altogether different closet, along with other straight men who can proudly say, "I love getting fucked in the ass!"

Prostate stimulation may take some getting used to. Make sure to give your partner helpful hints about what kinds of stimulation feel the best. Realize also that when some men have their ass stimulated, they may lose their erection; no one is exactly sure why this happens. Don't be alarmed if it happens to you or your partner. A loss of erection could signal a man's fear or anxiety about being penetrated, and you may want to check in with your partner if you sense some physical or emotional discomfort. However, a man may also be having the time of his life and still have a less than rock-hard cock. It's okay, it just means your body is more focused on your ass than your cock at the moment. It may not happen every time you are penetrated, or it may change as you become aroused. Worrying about your loss of erection is not going to help it return or help you to have a good time. Relax, and let it do whatever it wants to do.

As women try out the role of active penetrator, we can slip our tongues, fingers, and (rubber) cocks inside our male lovers' bodies, learning how to give and get pleasure in a brand-new way. Being on the other side of the dick is a chance for women to have their own revolution, too. We can see how the other half does it, and experience our power as women in a new way. Since our anorectal anatomy is so similar, all the tips and techniques you read about in this chapter apply to both women and men. You can use your mouth, your fingers, or an anal-sex toy to penetrate your man's ass. Some couples, however, like to experience their anal pleasure with a strap-on dildo.

Strap-On Sex Tips

For many reasons, strap-ons are a great way to experience anal penetration. Dildos and harnesses mean that you can have a hands-free fuck, and use your mitts for other things. People also like the closeness (of body and mind) that a strap-on affords partners during penetration. With a strap-on, a woman can put her whole body behind the penetration, and feel what it's like to shoot from the hip, so to speak.

Every single day that I worked at woman-owned sex-toy store Toys in Babeland, at least one straight couple bought a dildo and harness for her to fuck him. Remember "My First Pony," a sweet toy for little girls? Well, for all you adventurous couples, I recommend what I call "My first strap-on"—for the ride of both your lives. It's a slim silicone dildo, seven inches long with a 1¼-inch diameter (Toys in Babeland calls it "Mistress" and Good Vibrations calls it "Champ #1"), which I consider to be the best for virgin voyagers. Add a simple, functional harness of your choice and, of course, lots and lots of lube.

There is a growing selection of harnesses made of leather, vinyl, nylon webbing, and even denim; two of the best manufacturers of quality harnesses (who also do retail sales) are Stormy Leather in San Francisco and Aslan Leather in Toronto, Canada. Your choice of material depends on how you want your harness to look and how much money you want to spend.

Harnesses come in several styles, and your selection should depend on both function and aesthetics. (See illustration 8.) There is a basic triangle harness with one strap that fits between your legs; this harness tends to fit especially petite women the best. Because it fits like a G-string, the center strap rubs against your genitals, which may feel stimulating to some and annoying to others. There is a two-strapped harness with a triangle front which you wear like a jock strap; this style places the straps around your ass cheeks, leaving your vagina and ass easily accessible and free to be stimulated. People find that the two-strap harness tends to give them more control than the one strap model; the dildo moves around less and is easier to guide. Both of these triangle styles have a hole where you slip the dildo through, which rests against your pubic mound.

If you prefer something between you and the dildo, there is a two-strap harness with a piece of material behind the cock ring. This style (sometimes called the "Terra Firma" harness) also allows you to change the size of the cock ring, which is especially good if the dildo you are using is significantly smaller or larger than an average sized one. You also have a choice of fas-

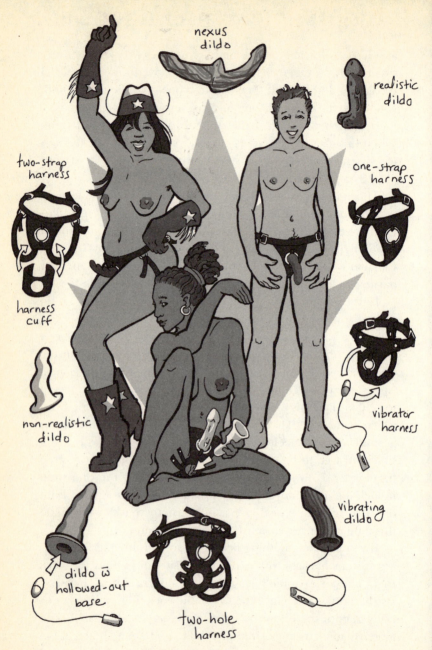

nexus dildo

realistic dildo

two-strap harness

one-strap harness

harness cuff

non-realistic dildo

vibrator harness

dildo w̄ hollowed-out base

vibrating dildo

two-hole harness

FIG. 8   STRAP-ON ANAL SEX

teners on your harness, either buckles or D-rings. There are plenty of other styles, including those made to fit plus-sized women. See what fits you best and is easiest for you to adjust.

You want to choose a harness that fits you well—the snugger and more secure the better. I recommend that you try a few different styles on before you buy them, or if you order from a catalog, see what the return policy is. The majority of dildos will fit in a standard harness, as long as there is a flared base and the dildo isn't excessively large. For beginning anal players, I would recommend a smaller dildo to start out.

As a woman doing the penetration, you should experiment with different positions. I know that the first few times I fucked someone in the ass with a strap-on, I had the person in traditional doggie-style position for several reasons. Doggie style gives you a clear view of the butthole, so you can see exactly what you're doing, and the position allows for a good angle of penetration toward the prostate. It's also an easy position to get your balance, establish a rhythm, and get some good thrusting going. So, you may want to start out that way, but you can also try missionary (usually with legs over the shoulders) or man-on-top.

Learning how to skillfully wield a strap-on takes practice and patience. If you feel like the dildo is moving around too much or doesn't feel secure, then your harness isn't tight enough and you should adjust it. In the beginning, you may want to guide the dildo with your hand, which will give you more control of exactly where it's going. When your partner is ready for penetration, be gentle and go slowly. Press the tip of the well-lubricated dildo against his opening, and have him come back on it. This may help him feel less vulnerable, and will reassure you that you're not hurting him. Once you are inside him, and he's ready for some movement, begin slowly. You want to establish a thrusting motion with your hips, one that feels good to him and won't tire you out too quickly.

Women can enjoy penetrating men on many different levels. The trust and intimacy between partners can feel especially heightened and very arousing. The naughty, taboo aspects of both anal sex and a woman with a dick can really get her motor going. The power she feels as the penetrating partner can also add to her fantasy and pleasure. Women, you'll be happy to know that strap-on anal sex also has the potential to be physically stimulating for you.

There are several opportunities for women to get a little action themselves while they are giving it to their guys. For some women, when the base of the dildo rubs against the clitoris and vagina, there is enough friction there to feel fantastic. There is a textured silicone square made by Dils for Does called "The Magic Carpet," which you wear between the dildo and your pussy; its bumps and grooves give you extra stimulation in all the right places. I also want to add a plug for dildos with balls. Some women don't choose a dildo with balls simply because they prefer a more nonrealistic style. However, balls do more than make it look real; they extend the base of the dildo and cover more surface area—which means more for you to rub up against. Think about it.

If you'd like to add a vibrator to the equation, you have several options. You could select a vibrating dildo, which will deliver vibration to both you and your partner. You could try to don a wearable vibrator beneath your harness, but this may be awkward and interfere with the harness being tight enough. A better idea is the "Buzz Me" harness made by Stormy Leather and equipped with a pocket for a small vibrating egg. Or Vixen Creations has several dildos, among them "Treasure Chest" and "Bobby Sue," with hollowed-out bases. Stick a vibrating egg in the base of the dildo, tuck the battery pack in the side of your harness, and you're ready for vibrating action, his and hers style!

Perhaps you want something inside you while you put something inside him; well, you can do that too. There are harnesses with two holes, one for the dildo to penetrate him with, another for a dildo pointing in your direction (made by Outrageous Cre-

Strap-On Sex Videos

- *Bend Over Boyfriend:* The first and only sex-instruction video all about women giving men anal pleasure. After a detailed anatomy lesson and hands-on demonstration by Carol Queen and Robert Morgan, two other couples try out their expert tips and techniques.

- *Bend Over Boyfriend 2: More Rockin', Less Talkin':* Focuses less on the educational details and turns its attention to five hot sex scenes of girls strappin' it on and stickin' it in.

- *Babes Ballin' Boys:* Very entertaining mainstream video series with porn stars.

ations and Stormy Leather). Stormy Leather makes a "harness cuff," which can transform a one hole harness into a two-hole harness. There are also double-headed dildos designed by Vixen and Tantus especially for one-hole harness use. The "Nexus" by Vixen is not an extra long jelly dong like you see in adult novelty stores. Instead, it's a two dildos-in-one package: you can have a dildo inside your vagina or your ass while simultaneously penetrating your partner. I just love sex-toy technology.

I *have never had two guys penetrate me at the same time, but I really want to do this. I think the idea of having two cocks in me—one in my pussy and one in my ass—would be an unbelievable feeling. However, this seems to be a hard thing to pull off. Do you have any tips on how to make this experience as pleasurable as possible?*

Congrats for being able to voice your fantasy out loud and tell your boyfriend. Some people think that it's just a very popular circus trick in porn, but there are real women who love to have both holes filled (and fucked) at once. My first piece of advice is that maybe the two of you should practice some double penetration before you invite a friend over. Begin at the beginning, with one well-lubed finger in each hole, and work your way up from there. Use lots and lots of lube, go slow, and see what kind of movement feels best.

When you are ready to graduate to something bigger, use a flexible vibrator or dildo in your ass as your boyfriend penetrates your vagina. Start out with both inside only part of the way, and gradually move farther as you feel ready. Communication is extremely important: you're testing the limits of your body, so make sure you give your man plenty of feedback about how it feels. Also realize that some women can easily and comfortably accommodate something of size in their pussy and in their ass. Others will take some effort, with lots of warm-up. But some women may not be able to do it at all, since double penetration really depends on your internal map, and if there's room for two. You are the one who will know best if it's possible, so make sure you're the one who's in charge and calling the shots. Work out the kinks on your dildo before you plan your threesome.

When you are ready to tackle two flesh cocks at once, again, use plenty of lube and go really slow. Depending on the size and height of all three of you, some positions will work better than others. You may want to straddle one man and have the other penetrate you from behind. Try to take one cock about halfway inside your pussy, then angle your body to take the other one in your ass. Both men should start with very shallow penetration, so you can get used to the feeling. Remember that porn stars make it look easy in adult movies, but they are seasoned professionals! You may be much more awkward your first time around.

BE YOUR OWN
FAIRY GODMOTHER!

Fantasy and Role-Playing

Fantasy can be an incredibly useful force in our lives, erotic and otherwise. Everyone has fantasies about sex and other erotic activities, but too many people are afraid to vocalize their secret thoughts. We fear that our lovers may question, criticize, ridicule, or reject us because of them. The myths and misinformation about certain sexual taboos contribute to this silence and sometimes prevent men and women from satisfying their curiosities. Some people feel so stifled by guilt, shame, or fear that they cannot even tap into what turns them on, let alone say it aloud.

Fantasies are a positive and powerful part of our lives; they can give us great insight into our deepest needs and fears. Give yourself permission to let your mind wander wherever it wants to as your hand wanders between your legs. See where a certain fantasy may take you during lovemaking with your partner. Nurture your fantasies, respect them, pay attention to them, even probe and question them—they may tell you surprising things about yourself.

Discovering Your Fantasies

One way to unearth your fantasies is to meditate, visualize, write in a journal, or do what it takes for you to get in touch with your inner self. You may want to make a list of what you thought about the last five times you masturbated, paying particular attention to the people, places, activities, or scenarios that really turned you on. Many people use their imagination when they pleasure themselves (and also when they are with a partner), and the images that come to mind can give you a window into your fantasies. Try reading an erotic story in a book or magazine, and see what arouses and excites you. Was it the dark alley where the two characters met? The sexy underwear the woman wore? The amazing blow job she gave? The way he talked dirty to her while he fucked her?

Likewise, watching movies—both adult and mainstream—is another method of tapping into your desires. (Read more about watching adult films in the next chapter.) What leading men or women turn you on and why? What's your favorite love scene in a movie and what about it really rocks your world? Erotic stories and films can be a great way to see your own desires written on the page or acted on the screen and articulated for you. In some cases, you might not have known that something really revved you up until you read about it or saw it. When people use erotica, they often discover fantasies they never even knew they had. Allow yourself to be open to new possibilities and ready for inspiration.

Opening Your Mouth

Once you're able to summon the words to describe what really floats your boat, consider sharing them with a partner. Sharing our sexual fantasies with a partner can deepen a sexual relationship and help us to better communicate. Too many times we keep secret desires from our partners because we're afraid to share them. Sometimes, we fear that our partner's reaction will be negative: he or she will think we're weird or perverted. The fear of being shamed by a lover is very strong and often keeps us silent. Many of us feel that if we say something out loud, it will change the way our lover feels about us; specifically, it will make them love us less or not love us at all. These are serious feelings that can feel overwhelming and devastating. Sometimes, these feelings are simply a reflection of the shame and guilt we feel for having the fantasies in the first place, and they aren't a realistic assessment of how our partners might react. But if you and your partner are very different in your comfort levels with sexual experimentation, you may actually be correct in your assumptions and expectations about his or her reaction. Only you can gauge your relationship, but try to look at the situation objectively and see that maybe your own fears are getting in the way of voicing your fantasies.

If (and hopefully when) you've decided to share a fantasy with a partner, I find that a good way to do it is in a neutral, nonsexual context. In other words, lovemaking may not be the best time to tell your partner one of the fantasies that has been swimming around your head—it can feel too threatening to the other person, maybe too overwhelming, and both of you might feel too vulnerable at that moment to react in any useful way. It can also bring a perfectly hot encounter to a screeching halt if, in fact, your partner does have some negative feelings or issues about what you just said.

It's a better idea to create a safe space where both people will feel comfortable and a dialogue on the subject can begin. This also means that bringing it up at work, at the movies, or at your parents' house just isn't fair; you need to be alone and have the opportunity to talk openly and honestly without fear that someone will overhear you or that you're on a time limit. If you're nervous, you can preface your conversation by saying something like "I want to talk about something with you and I want you to have an open mind about it. Remember that I love you and it's difficult for me to tell you this, but I want to because I want our sexual relationship to be as full as possible. I want to share this with you because I am hoping that it might give you some insight into me, it might bring us closer, and help us be even more intimate and connected." Of course, this is just an example. Say what's in your heart and do it in your own words.

A fantasy doesn't necessarily have to be an elaborate one to cause you anxiety about bringing it up with your lover. You may want to try something new—it might be anal sex, bondage, using a sex toy, or trying out a new technique. I hope you realize by now that I am a very direct person, and I am all about cutting to the chase and just saying it; so in general, I advocate being as direct as possible with people, especially when it comes to sex. However, that said, if you honestly have no idea how your partner feels about something and you want to simply gauge his or her take on it, you could employ a less direct approach. Instead of raising an issue for you personally, you can bring it up as a more hypothetical situation. For example: "I read about a workshop on bondage being given in our area . . . [pause, giving your partner a chance to say something in response]." Or: "I read in a magazine about female ejaculation . . ." These general, open-ended statements are nonthreatening and give your lover an opportunity to respond without being directly confronted.

If your partner reveals something about your sex life, use it as a chance to start a dialogue and probe deeper. For example, a man at one of my workshops once said, "My girlfriend and I have been together for five years and recently she told me she wants to spice things up in our sex life. I don't want her getting bored, but how do I keep it hot for her?" I told him that the first thing he should do is ask her exactly what she wants. She may have had some ideas and fantasies already in her head and was just waiting for him to inquire about them. Asking her directly is always better than guessing.

In general, people (especially women) appreciate when they

know that you have thought about a romantic encounter and put time and energy into planning one. So, whether you surprise her one night with candles, music, and a sensual massage or flowers, a bottle of wine, and an erotic video, she'll feel desired and special. Making time for each other in our hectic lives of work, family, and plenty of stress is difficult, but so important. Maybe you have to plan a weekend somewhere else to get away from it all, a time when you can focus solely on one another and reconnect in an intimate way. I am also a big fan of dating, even for long-term couples: asking her out, picking her up (even if you live together), dressing for each other, and going out on the town. Sometimes a fantasy is just about making time for each other.

Once you've been able to share your fantasies with your partner, you may want to transform them into reality. Creating a fantasy for you and your partner to share can be simple; it just takes some planning, a dash of creativity, and both of your imaginations.

A New Perspective

Sometimes, the easiest way to get a new view of the world is to simply roll over. Trying out an old trick in a new position may be just the thing you need to alter your perspective. Don't underestimate the power of changing places. Besides just shifting your "routine," different positions can produce new physical sensations; for example, maybe you've never tried spooning before (lying side by side, facing each other or the same direction), and you discover that it's the perfect angle for penetrating her vagina and stimulating her clitoris simultaneously. Or maybe you find that anal penetration while you're on top of him lets you control the action and depth of penetration. The ways in which we position our bodies in relation to one another can also create different dynamics between partners. If you want to feel as if you are surrendering to your lover, try putting your ass in the air, with your head and shoulders down on the bed. By contrast, face-to-face lovemaking, where you look into each other's eyes, can enhance the intimate connection between you.

In some cases, a fantasy may involve a sexual activity you've never tried before together—such as anal sex, bondage, or using a vibrator. In this case, you need a few items—lube for the anal sex, something to tie him up with for the bondage, or a vibrator. Buying the item together may be a fun way to get the ball rolling. Beyond equipment, you need desire and a date to do the deed and you're all set. Planning a date lets you take advantage of the pleasure of anticipation. If you are trying something brand-new and want to read about it beforehand, I encourage research. There are great books on all kinds of specific subjects in which you can find useful information about how to do it, and hopefully, how to do it well. There may be an instructional video on the particular topic you're interested in or even a workshop given in your area (see the Resource Guide for some suggestions). Just like anything else you're doing for the first time, be gentle with yourself. Have the patience to explore this new terrain, and don't expect perfection the first time around. Bring plenty of love, desire, and enthusiasm to the task, set realistic expectations and goals, and remember that your virgin voyage doesn't have to be the best ever. That's what makes this fantasy so much fun: practice, practice, practice!

Stripping for Your Lover

For example, say you'd like to perform an erotic striptease for your lover. First of all, congratulations on being so brave! Not everyone has the guts to explore their exhibitionist side and perform for their lover. Like other kinds of fantasies, think of your striptease as a piece of theater. What will you wear? I suggest lots of layers—not the Montana-in-winter kind, but you should have enough different pieces on to make the stripping worthwhile. You need to select a suitable piece of music, and that totally depends on you: what songs make you feel your most sexy? Whether it's Madonna or Marvin Gaye, you want a tune that's going to put you and your lover in the mood.

Being the anal retentive planner that I am, I am all about practicing. Now, this doesn't mean that a spontaneous strip cannot be just as sensuous and effective as that well-choreographed and rehearsed little number. But I always say, if you're gonna do it, do it well. Try out your moves in front of a mirror. Get comfortable with the music so you know it by heart. Also become well acquainted with the business of taking off your clothes in a seductive and graceful way—trust me, sometimes it's not as easy as it looks!

Set realistic expectations for yourself, and do not attempt to transform into Nina Hartley overnight; be yourself and make the most of your own assets, whatever they are. If you can actually dance, go for it; if you can't, just fake it. The most important thing to remember about stripping is to do every single move about ten times slower than you think you need to: work every single second for all it's worth. Effort and enthusiasm really go a long way. Chances are that your lover will be so flattered and turned on that the little details will be forgotten when you fall into his (or her!) arms.

The Main Course

A fantasy common among lots of different people is to incorporate exotic, sensual, or simply delicious foods into a sexual encounter. Food and sex seem like such an obvious and complementary pair, since eating can be incredibly sensuous in and of itself. This fantasy is fairly easy to execute as well.

One of the first times I tried out my food fantasy, my lover and I went shopping (separately) for treats. Then, we each took turns blindfolding the other person, feeding the secret food to each other, and trying to guess what had passed between our lips. The indescribable texture of gummi worms is what stumped me. From sweet truffles, berries, and cake morsels to juicy peaches, plums, and melons, feeding a lover can feel sexy and decadent. Perhaps you'd like to eat something *off* of your partner's body; that's when chocolate sauce, whipped cream, honey, and caramel are easy to drip on and fun to lick up. To add an extra sensation to this version of food play, drag an ice pop along her inner thighs or heat up the hot fudge before you spread it on his chest. Foods like oysters, avocados, artichokes, and chiles are aphrodisiacs all by themselves, and they may inspire sex by being consumed before, rather than during, the activities.

Whatever foods you choose, make sure you think about how to clean up before you start rolling around in chocolate on the white sheets. When it comes to anything sugary or fruity, putting it near her pussy is sexy, but putting it *in* her pussy could produce a yeast infection, so be careful.

Location, Location, Location

Some fantasies are all about where sex happens—at the office, in a public bathroom, in a park, in a car, on an airplane, at a sleazy motel. The location, whether public, exotic, risky, or out of the ordinary, is part of what makes you want to rip each other's clothes off. For this fantasy to work, all you really need to do is find the place, and you're halfway there.

Use a little bit of creativity if the actual location you're after just isn't accessible. For instance, if you want to get a little nooky in the Oval Office, try doing it at *your* office (preferably after hours, and with the door locked). With an American flag on the wall, you'll never know the difference, and you can still feel patriotic. Maybe you want to relive your first date and get busy in the back row of a movie theater; the only problem is they tore down the theater to build condos. Find another cinema with the same vibe as your original—you won't know the difference when the lights go down and you both reach for the popcorn.

If you're going to bring your roll in the hay to somewhere public, just make sure it's a place that's actually safe to have sex. There's a fine line to walk between pleasure and danger when it comes to public sex. The idea of getting caught is mostly likely part of the turn-on for a lot of people with public-sex fantasies; however, you need to be sensible when choosing your site. Scout it before you bring your sweetie there; spontaneous public sex can be fun but can also put you in an very embarrassing situation. Once you've found the perfect spot, be sure to dress the part—skirts and no panties are a plus, pants you can easily unzip are too.

Public bathrooms meant for one person are fairly easy to pull off or, if you have the choice of multiple stalls, pick the extralarge handicapped-accessible one. If you've always wanted to get down under the bleachers during a football game, why not do a test-run when no one's playing the field? It might be just as fun.

Fantasy Role-Playing

Role-playing is a fun, sexy way to explore situations outside your normal, everyday existence. One of the questions people ask me most often about role-playing is: how do I begin? Think of it as putting on your own private play. You need characters: do you want to be a real person, a historical figure, a celebrity, or a fictional character? Maybe you want to be yourself, but in a different scenario. You may also want costumes or props to help put you in the fantasy. What about dialogue, a plot or story line? Role-playing can involve as few or as many accoutrements as you want, just don't forget the most important ingredient: imagination.

In one way, role-playing is your chance to be a kid again—to be carefree, uninhibited, and ready to play in a make-believe world. Think back to a time when you'd say what came to mind without fear of embarrassment and you'd follow your dreams wherever they took you. Capture your kidlike wonder and know that this time there are some significant differences: playing doctor can go all the way; your game of cops and robbers has a blatant erotic charge; and the Cinderella fairy tale involves a girl with dominatrix sisters and a prince with a shoe fetish.

Who Do You Want to Be?

When some people fantasize, they imagine themselves as other people, distinctive characters in an erotic drama. First, ask yourself who you'd like to be and who you want your partner to be. For instance, you may want to draw from classic and colorful historical figures. Are you drawn to the romance and nobility of King Arthur and Guinevere? Does the legend of Robin Hood and Maid Marion make you wet? You might also imagine yourselves to be real, larger-than-life celebrities like Joe DiMaggio and Marilyn Monroe, Bogie and Bacall, or Tommy Lee and Pamela Anderson. Sometimes characters that movie stars portray are even more appealing, and lend themselves to titillating sexual scenarios—Han Solo and Princess Leia, Rhett Butler and Scarlett O'Hara, Romeo and Juliet. Fantasies are all about suspending disbelief and using your imagination. If you can dream it, chances are you can make it happen.

You don't have to pressure yourself to be too specific either; you can choose simple archetypes and flesh out specific characters later. Sometimes, all you need are two roles—like sergeant and cadet, boss and secretary, or pimp and prostitute. The powerful, erotic dynamic built into the roles may be plenty of food for thought and all you need to bring your characters to life. How do you figure out which role is for you? When you watch an old silent film, are you the damsel in distress on the railroad

Erotic Roles

- Boss and Secretary

- Teacher and Student

- Truck Driver and Hitchhiker

- Doctor and Patient

- Police Officer and Criminal

- Guard and Prisoner

- Quarterback and Cheerleader

- Sergeant and Cadet

- Client and Prostitute

- Master and Slave

tracks or the rescuing hero? In a Clint Eastwood movie, are you the good-guy cowboy or the bad-guy outlaw? In a naughty-schoolboy fantasy, which one of you is most likely to wield the ruler?

You can also select a particular scenario you find sexy, and meditate on it until you "find" your character. It could be the regiment of boot camp, the desperation of a deserted island, or the harshness of a prison. You can be a captured spy being inter-rogated and defiled by your unrelenting enemy captor. Many people have fantasies about having anonymous sex with com-plete strangers; I know a couple who regularly act this one out by arranging to meet somewhere and pretending they don't know one another. Then they go home together and have pas-sionate sex all night. Maybe you want to relive an important moment in your life like losing your virginity. Losing one's inno-cence can be very sexually and emotionally charged, and reen-

Sexy Scenarios

The First Time: Losing your virginity to an older, wiser, more experienced lover who instructs and initiates you.

Kidnapped: You've been snatched off the street, now you'll be interrogated by your captor and made to sexually service him/her.

The Stranger: Pretend you've never met each other, and pick up your lover on the bus, at the grocery store, or in a bar; take him to your place for some anonymous sex.

acting the first time can be really hot. Playing the naive novice who needs to be shown what to do and how to do it may appeal to you most. Or, as the wiser, more experienced deflowerer, you are in a position to teach and train your partner, and perhaps guide him or her in a way that you cannot outside of role playing. Or perhaps you are both teenagers fumbling around, excitedly exploring each other's bodies for the very first time.

Forbidden Fantasies

In some of our fantasies, we not only want to be another person, but someone of a different gender. Some people who play with gender also get great pleasure out of cross-dressing. Do not be alarmed by gender-play fantasies; in most cases, they do not represent a deep need to actually change your sex or a case of gender dysphoria (where a person feels like his or her gender does not match his or her body). Many people simply want to experience what it might be like to button up a shirt the other way for a change, and all that comes with it. These fantasies can be especially difficult to bring up with a partner. People with gender-play fantasies can feel very vulnerable and might fear that their partners will suspect they are gay or transgendered.

Hopefully, you have a partner who respects and listens to you, and who won't judge any fantasy of yours, including one of gender play.

Some of the most taboo and forbidden fantasies can also be the hottest. An example that leaps to mind is role-playing an intergenerational sex scene, like an older woman and a teenage boy or a mature man and a young girl. For some people, the power dynamic between the two roles is undeniable and this "age play" is very sexually charged and powerful. For others, it is just too taboo to ever turn them on. Other taboo themes include forced sex or rape, pedophilia, sex with animals, or incest.

A word of advice: toss your political correctness aside for a moment and remember these are fantasies. They might not jibe with your social conscience, your political beliefs, or your humanitarian ideals. Go easy on yourself. Just because they may turn you on with your partner doesn't mean you condone them in real life. You may get off when the boss does the secretary and her job is at stake, but it doesn't mean you support sexual harassment. The whole idea is to suspend reality and follow your mind, your heart, and your libido to wherever they take you.

That said, if you and your partner agree to enact one of these fantasies, be prepared. Because taboos can be highly charged emotionally, people can react in a variety of different ways. Intense feelings of fear, hurt, sadness, anger, and more may come up and you need to be ready to support each other if a particular fantasy pushes your buttons in ways you couldn't have predicted.

Getting into Character

Once you've decided who you want to be, in order to get into character, you may need a costume; remember, this can be as elaborate or as simple as you want and your budget allows. If you imagine yourself a dominatrix, you could go all the way and spend a chunk of change on a fabulous latex catsuit, a menacing mask, domineering high heels, and a selection of exquisite torture devices. Or maybe all you need is a great pair of killer patent-leather boots, the kind you wouldn't normally wear. Once you slip those beauties on, you become Mistress, and your lover becomes sex slave for the evening. It could be that one partner's costume works to get both of you into your roles. All I need to become a queen is a crown; once that shiny symbol is resting on my head, my partner automatically becomes a loyal subject. Maybe you need your lover to don the uniform of a delivery guy or the meter reader to become the bored-but-horny housewife on the other side of the door. You may need a wig and a white dress to be Marilyn Monroe. Whether it's a baseball cap or a full-body costume, clothing helps you create your character.

Perhaps clothes do not make the man in your case (maybe you're both wearing nothing at all!), but one or two props can really set the scene. These can be easy-to-find household items that, used in the right context, transform into highly erotic objects—like a tongue depressor and a thermometer for the age-old favorite "playing doctor" or a ruler and notebook for the strict teacher and naughty student just dying to come out and play. For me, a football and pompoms can help live out that cheerleader fantasy I've always had.

Quiet on the Set!

In keeping with the theatrical theme, you need to think about your set. Sometimes location can make or break a fantasy. Be realistic and creative. If you can't sneak a quickie at the office, live out your boss-and-secretary fantasy on a desk at home. If you want to relive the fateful affair from *Titanic,* why not borrow a friend's sailboat? If your lover has always wanted you to strip for him, you don't need to rent an entire gentleman's club; just a sexy outfit, dim lights, and some sultry music will do the trick (lap dance optional, of course, for which you need a chair).

One of my absolute favorite places to have sex is in a hotel room, because it represents neutral territory. For one thing, no one knows you are there, so you can't get phone calls, faxes, or e-mail; the stresses of your everyday life can be left outside. None of our "stuff" (both physical and emotional) is there either. When you walk through the door into that room, usually generic and uncluttered, you can be whomever you want to be in that moment. A perfect setting for fantasies, hotels also vary greatly in their potential for different scenarios: the decadent opulence of an expensive luxury hotel; the over-the-top heart-shaped bed in a hotel for lovers; the seedy, sleazy, rent-by-the-hour motel off the highway; or the simplicity of a midpriced motel. A bed, a bathroom, and endless possibilities.

If you are going to live out your fantasy at home, one way to make it seem less familiar is to make the bed differently (try brand-new white sheets for the hospital scene or satin sheets for the princess and her servant). You could light candles, burn incense, or use an aromatherapy oil to give the room a different feel and smell. You also may want to take fabric, scarves, or sheets and cover things like a computer, the television set, the telephone, and anything else that reminds you of your real life. These everyday items can distract from the fantasy at hand. A cleverly placed piece of furniture (the interrogation chair) or prop (the baseball glove) can also serve to transform a familiar room into the set of your own erotic drama.

These are only a few examples of how to use the theatrical concepts of characters, plots, costumes, props, and settings to help tap into your role-playing fantasies and figure out how to re-create them. There are obviously millions of others—give yourself permission to let your mind go wild. And remember, the two of you are the directors and the stars: you make the rules, you set any restrictions, you run the show.

If you and your partner are really into fantasy and role-playing, you may feel that the planning of the fantasies takes away from the spontaneity of your sex. One way to keep yourselves guessing and even surprise each other on occasion is to create a "Fantasy Keeper." The Fantasy Keeper can be any container—a jar or a box or even a small drawer—just make sure it's private. You don't need your kids, the baby-sitter, or an inquisitive friend stumbling on it. Each time you come up with a fantasy, write it down on a piece of paper, with as much detail and information as possible, and put it in the Fantasy Keeper. Then, each of you can draw a fantasy randomly and surprise your partner one night.

Irreconcilable Differences?

Your fantasy may not go over very well with your lover, and you need to be prepared for that possibility. Instead of throwing in the towel completely, first try discussing it. It's okay to have a dialogue about your fantasy, but it's unacceptable to try to convince or coerce your partner into doing something she or he does not want to do. Ask your partner why a particular fantasy does not appeal to him or her. Have you had a negative experience in the past? Have you tried it already and know you don't like it? Do you have fears about pain, discomfort, injury, or health concerns? Do you have issues because you think the fantasy is kinky or weird? Does the fantasy seem to contradict your spiritual beliefs? Does it push your buttons or raise issues for you that you'd rather not explore in a sexual context? These are just a few questions you can gently pose to your lover. Having an honest exchange in which both parties feel safe to voice their feelings can bring you greater insight into what makes your partner tick sexually. It may not make your fantasy happen, but it may bring you a better understanding of each other.

Often, people have preconceived notions or misinformation about certain sexual activities; they simply need to air their concerns, and get some concrete information, before they can move beyond their fear of doing something different. I've found this is often the case with anal sex. When a man brings up the subject to his partner, sometimes a woman's rejection of it is based on the fear of experiencing pain, a story she heard about how it can damage the rectum, or other myths about this taboo sexual subject. When men reassure women that it can be pain-free and pleasurable for them and when they counter the myths with valid information, many women feel more open to exploring their back doors.

In some cases, you may be able to modify your fantasy in order for it to appeal to both partners. As long as you approach the idea with love and respect for yourself and your partner, there may be a way for you both to meet somewhere in the middle. With a creative imagination and a willingness to be satisfied with a different "version" of your fantasy, you can create something that works for both of you.

In my experience of teaching sex workshops nationwide, I've found that one of the most popular fantasies among men is to have a threesome with their partner and another woman. Unfortunately for them, most of their female partners aren't so gung-ho about the ménage à trois. (If you are up to making two become three, then definitely check out my advice about multiple-partner arrangements in the Q&A at the end of this chapter.) The mistake men make with this fantasy is wanting to go all the way and thus missing the opportunity to explore a range of different ways to make this fantasy happen. Girls, I don't mean to encourage men everywhere to pressure you into a *Three's Company*–style romp; instead, I want to give a concrete example about how to make the fantasy work for both of you.

Ladies: so your man wants to have a three-way, but you're not into it. You still have a few options, if you are willing to compromise. This is basically about getting to the core of what about the fantasy turns him on and making some changes to accommodate the needs and desires of you and your lover. One solution is to go together to a strip club for a lap dance. If he's never been to one, get a recommendation for a place that is couples-friendly and where you will feel most comfortable. Girls: You should select the dancer for your lap dance and feel free to interact with her as much as you feel comfortable with (many clubs actually have a hands-off policy, so you may not be able to touch her even if you want to). Your guy can watch as the two of you have an erotic encounter, but you don't actually have to have sex with another woman, which may not be your thing. If you find such a club too public, try a peep show with booths and dancers behind glass for more privacy. You may have less direct contact with the dancer, but that may be easier for you.

If you'd rather have no physical contact at all, you have several options. One is for the both of you to call a phone-sex line and have an erotic chat with a female phone-sex operator where you verbally play out the fantasy. This is a very safe option and still may do the trick. Or you could venture onto the Web to an adult site with live chat and live interactions with women. Equally safe but probably more expensive, cybersex is more visual than the phone call and may appeal to the computer geeks out there. Perhaps he's got a favorite dirty story about a threesome from a magazine or book that he can read to you before bedtime. You can always rent an adult video with some "hot girl/girl action" and watch it together. Or for those of you with more enterprising and vocal men on your hands, encourage him to let his imagination run wild and whisper a tale to you about his fantasy while you're making love. As these suggestions illustrate, with some ingenuity, you can bring almost any fantasy to life in some form or another. The key is to listen to your partner and come up with a solution that works for you both. Also know when to let a fantasy remain a fantasy out of respect for your lover's boundaries and limits.

When delving into the world of fantasies, you still need to keep in mind that there are some fantasies destined to remain just that—fantasies. We like them and get off on them, but we don't want them to actually happen. For example, you may not want to be jumped by a hooded stranger in a strange place (or re-create that scene with your lover), but the thought of it sends you over the edge when you masturbate. In real life, you don't have any desire to have sex for money, but in your head, the images you come up with make your body tingle. The one thing that makes you soak your panties is thinking about a snake slithering inside you, but in actuality, no boa constrictor is going anywhere near your private parts. And that's okay. The most important thing is that you are having fantasies and they are fueling your pleasure, whether alone or with a partner.

Q&A

My wife and I are thinking we may want to include other people in our relationship. Some of our friends have relationships they call "open" or "polyamorous." What exactly is polyamory?

Polls show that 40 to 60 percent of people cheat on their spouses at least once, and that half of all marriages end in divorce. The nature of our relationships and of the institution of marriage are shifting. So it doesn't surprise me that you are interested in polyamory, because more and more people share your interest in expanding their relationships. Polyamory is a catch-all term for many different relationships that fall outside the traditional, sexually faithful, two-person model we call monogamy. Some people see polyamory as a postmillennial antidote to chronic serial monogamy that includes an abundance of cheating, embarrassment, deception, scandal, separation, and divorce. Many polyamorous couples practice nonmonogamy—the partners are emotionally committed to one another, but their relationship isn't sexually exclusive. Some poly people have multiple partners with whom they have both sexual and emotional/love relationships. Some polyamorous couples expand to become a triad or a group.

Polyamory for couples requires honesty, communication, boundaries, mutual respect, and rules—rules based on your individual relationship, desires, needs, and goals, rules that everyone can agree on, rules you need to stick to. You may decide that having the occasional ménage à trois to spice things up is okay by both of you. Or you may allow each other to have sex-only partners as long as you two remain the primary relationship. Your rules are whatever you need (no sleepovers? no anal sex? no blondes?) to feel secure, sane, and satisfied. I know one polyamorous couple that comes to the table as a package deal: if you want to have sex with him, you have to do her, too. Another duo bases their sanctioned dalliances on geography; when either or both are out of town, they have free reign to do the nasty with whomever they choose. While in the same zip code, they remain true blue. A rad bisexual couple works the gender angle. She's allowed to dabble with other girls, but he's the only XY in her equation. He can have all the man-on-man action he wants, but must remain loyal to one and only one woman—her.

If you are interested in getting some guidelines, read the books *The Ethical Slut: A Guide to Infinite Sexual Possibilities* (don't let the name scare you, it's very useful and down to earth) and *Polyamory: The New Love Without Limits*. The magazine *Loving More* (www.lovemore.com) has a wealth of information on the subject and celebrates alternative arrangements of all kinds. While it may seem reminiscent of seventies free love without the drugs, polyamory today encompasses a greater consciousness of safer sex and everyone's feelings and boundaries than it did in the days of wife swapping and key parties. It's a surefire way to challenge your sexual and emotional boundaries and explore your feelings about jealousy and possessiveness. If you were actually allowed to stray within the confines of your relationship—the illicit naughtiness of an affair no longer present—would it still be desirable? Could you live with the knowledge that your partner was fucking someone else but still loved you? Polyamory is not a tool to avoid issues in your marriage, it's not an excuse to act out irresponsibly, and it's not for everyone. It takes just as much work as monogamy, and probably more honesty. The sneers *slut, swinger,* and *sex addict* may be vaulted your way by others, but check the source—they're probably just jealous.

8

STROKE BOOKS, SKIN MAGAZINES, AND BLUE MOVIES

Adding Erotica to Sex

Erotica Versus Pornography

What is the difference between erotica and pornography? No one has been able to answer that question definitively, and when you ask, everyone's got a different opinion. One porn fan put it this way: "Basically, if I like it, it's wonderful, life-affirming erotica. If you like it and I don't, it's cheap, sleazy porn."[18] I know someone who thinks the sole difference is in the lighting; if it's brightly and badly lit, it's got to be porn, but if it's got soft, artistic, or moody lighting, it's erotica. Others say erotica is expensive, tasteful, and highbrow, whereas pornography is cheap, lewd, and base. Or erotica is literary, intelligent, thoughtful, politically correct—if flowery metaphors are present, it's erotica—whereas porn is illiterate, stupid, crude, misogynist—if you hear the word *cock* or *cunt,* it's porn.

The age-old debate of erotica versus pornography, quite frankly, bores me. For one thing, the distinction between the two is based on economics even more than personal tastes. Representations of sex printed on expensive paper or hanging in museums are erotica, while the same thing found on a street in an disreputable neighborhood or announced in tawdry neon is porn. You get the idea. In critiquing the false distinction, Laurence O'Toole called erotica an "acceptable level of sexual expression," meaning, of course, that porn is *un*acceptable.[19] Differences between erotica and pornography are based on money, socioeconomic class, politics, culture, and, yes, personal taste, but far be it for me to judge if anyone has any.

Throughout this chapter and the entire book, I use the two terms interchangeably. I render no judgment on one or the other—they are identical in my eyes. To be honest, I used the term erotica in the chapter title simply so I wouldn't scare some of you off. I wanted to at least get you this far, which I hope I have, to realize that *porn* is not a bad word. Like *bitch* and *pussy* and *dyke,* let's reclaim it, so it's no longer dirty. Well, okay, maybe it's a little bit dirty . . .

Dirty Stories and Stroke Books

The written word—from no-nonsense stroke books to literary erotica—can be incredibly sexy. Lots of women tend to appreciate a story, characters, context, and emotional resonance to go with their fucking, and plenty of men are capable of lusting after writing as well.

There was a time when all you could find in the way of written erotica were inexpensive mass-market paperbacks. Several publishers have kept anonymous classics in print—titles like *Man with a Maid, Confessions of a Concubine,* and *Initiation Rites.* Although written decades ago, their smutty prurience stands the test of time. These cut-to-the-sex paperback novels are still available from publishers like Black Lace, Blue Moon, Nexus, and Masquerade Books. Many of them lack good writing, editing, and packaging, but there are a few gems out there and their compact size also makes them perfect for one-handed reading.

In the last two decades, the field of erotic writing has exploded and produced erotic novels and erotica anthologies that represent, inspire, and arouse people of all walks of life. Small presses and mainstream publishers have all gotten in on the act and published plenty of erotic books; in fact, there is such a variety available that you should be able to find something to suit your needs and tastes whatever they may be.

If you want to sample well-crafted tales of all different sexual orientations and proclivities, get one of the annual editions of Susie Bright's *Best American Erotica;* they are chock-full of superbly written erotica that runs the gamut of sexual orientations and activities. For erotica written by and for women, try the *Herotica* or *Best Women's Erotica* series. There are also gay and lesbian erotic books. Most erotica books are available through women's bookstores, adult and sex-toy stores, gay and lesbian bookstores, and online booksellers. They are also popping up more and more at chain bookstores, usually in the sexuality, anthology, or erotica sections.

You can use dirty stories and books to masturbate with, either by yourself or with a partner. Try reading a favorite story to your lover at bedtime and see what ideas it gives you; often an element of a story—a particular activity, scorching dirty talk, or a sexy scenario—can lead both of you to try something new. Erotic fiction may even inspire you to write your own story, starring the two of you; share the story with the other person, and maybe you can bring it to life. Reading erotica to your partner can also be an opportunity for you to share a personal fantasy; it may feel less scary to tell a story that represents the fantasy, rather than saying it outright. Later, you can tell your sweetie why that story really turned you on.

Skin Magazines

There is a prevailing notion that men are aroused only by sexually explicit material that is visual (and they cannot appreciate something more intellectual or literary) and women are not aroused by images, but instead prefer more cerebral, written works of erotica. The reality, of course, lies somewhere in between. Some women like pictures, some words, some both, and the same goes for men. Magazines often provide the best of both worlds, combining sexy fiction with spicy pictorials.

The most widely available porn magazines—popular titles like *Playboy, Penthouse,* and *Hustler* and dozens of others—are targeted toward men, and the images usually reflect their gender-slanted marketing strategy: airbrushed, tanned women with "perfect" bodies and big breasts (very often courtesy of plastic surgery). That doesn't mean that women cannot appreciate them. A well-known lesbian editor I know told me that before there were any authentic lesbian porn magazines, she used to keep *Penthouse* under the bed and drool over the girl/girl pictorials. These mainstream magazines have always enjoyed female subscribers. You don't need to be bisexual to appreciate looking at naked chicks, or even get off on them, so keep that in mind before dismissing them right off the bat. Many glossy skin mags—often those touting themselves as "hard-core" (which only means that they show penetration in their pictures) feature couples having sex. These may interest you more if the girls alone don't do anything for you. *Penthouse* also publishes other magazines more focused on stories and erotic confessionals (with a lot less photography) called *Penthouse Forum, Penthouse Letters,* and *Penthouse Variations,* which couples may like better. There are dozens of other adult magazines, from *High Society* and *Barely Legal* to *Oui* and *Perfect 10,* but for women readers they're going to be pretty hit or miss. Overall, mainstream skin mags can be pretty blatant about objectifying women and pretty lame when it comes to women's pleasure, so if that bothers you or your partner, then these magazines are probably not for you.

Playgirl features nude pictorials of men and is the only mainstream porn magazine specifically for women. *Playgirl* has basically taken the formula of *Playboy* and inserted men in place of women, which I am not convinced is the best way to go about making a women's porn magazine. Some women really appreciate having their own mag, while others don't find pictures of naked guys enough to stimulate their libidos.

There is another genre of magazine that tends to be more literary or "alternative," and often bills itself as erotica. Most of the publications in this group are underfunded (with a few exceptions), so don't expect glossy paper, color photos, or widespread distribution. Publishers of this kind of magazine often take a more thoughtful, less explicit approach, producing a softer, more artistic look at sex. Or they see sexuality in more radical and political terms. Through fiction, poetry, photography, and illustrations, readers can see new worlds beyond the genital close-ups and jerk-off stories of traditional porn. Many in this category have ceased publication in the last few years (titles like *Libido, Paramour,* and *Yellow Silk*), but some lesser-known erotic zines are still around, including *Black Sheets, Blue Blood,* and *EIDOS.* A few new titles have also come on the market, including *Nerve, Blue Food,* and *Zaftig.* While the mainstream glossies are relatively easy to find, look for the more obscure titles in adult and sex-toy stores, alternative bookstores, or online.

Looking at erotic photography is obviously a wonderful addition to solo or mutual masturbation. One way to incorporate this kind of porn into sex is for one or both of you to create a story to go with a photo or pictorial. Name the characters, explain the situation they're in, and spin a tale that's original, seductive, and playful. Your story can take on a life of its own and inspire the two if you. Pictures may also generate ideas of things you'd like to try with a partner. If there is a particular photo that represents a new position, an erotic setting, or a sexual activity you've always wanted to try, you can use the image to *show* rather than tell your lover about your desire.

Cybersmut

Some of the best visual and written erotica that's intelligent, funny, sexy, outrageous, unique, and arousing can be found on the Internet. Some Web sites cater specifically to a mainstream (predominantly) male audience, mostly offering downloadable hard-core images. Others feature erotic stories, photos, and other content that appeals to women, literary smut readers, or fans of fetish porn. Some sex sites attempt to cover sex from several different angles—with interviews, essays, how-tos, and news stories. The maverick spirit of the Web has also spawned dozens of homemade, amateur porn Web sites. Unique to the Web are some interesting interactive opportunities. Many people take advantage of the anonymity of the Web to have online cybersex in chat rooms. There are also streaming adult-video clips, voyeuristic Web cams, full-length adult features on demand, and live, interactive video feeds where you can chat with someone and have her or him act out a fantasy for you. New sites come online every day, others disappear without warning, and new technology is being developed even as I write this. A select list of URLs would be outdated by the time this book is published, but a good place to start is in some of your favorite print publications or a search engine.

The Web provides stories and images that you can use in the same ways you would the printed materials. In addition to giving you new ideas and concrete information about sex, the Internet can be a unique resource for sexual communication with your partner. On the Web, whether it's through e-mail or live chat, you can communicate with a lover in a totally different medium. You may be able to express a desire more easily and comfortably through an e-mail message than you'd be able to do face-to-face.

Whether you live together or in different cities, you can have cybersex online. You may try out some of your role-playing ideas through e-mail or chat, and sharpen your dirty-talk skills. When you log on, you really can be whomever you choose, and this freedom may be just what you need to play out a particular fantasy. The Internet can also be a creative, safe way to do things you might not do in "real life." For example, a three-way in cyberspace can feel less threatening, but still help you achieve the fantasy you want.

Blue Movies

Of all the different types of erotica, videos are among the most sexually explicit. Porn videos are also the most controversial of all erotica, since feminists, religious right wingers, and others have long argued that porn is sick, obscene, exploitative, misogynist, or downright evil. These debates have made their mark on mainstream popular consciousness, and they often leave both women and men feeling divided or guilty about their enjoyment of pornography. Certainly, there is plenty of porn that many people do find offensive, degrading to women, or immoral. However, there is also a diverse array of videos that people can enjoy for a variety of reasons.

When people think of porn, they may picture men in sleazy booths popping quarters into a machine to watch people fucking on-screen. But thanks to cable television and the invention of the VCR, you can enjoy porn in the comfort and privacy of your own home. Like other forms of erotica, adult videos may help you get off while masturbating. Some people simply use porn to be entertained and aroused, and to help them slip into a fantasy world wholly different from their own. Others need to be able to relate to the characters or stories to be turned on. There are plenty of ways to incorporate porn videos into your sex life. You can watch them with your partner as an appetizer; it can put both of you in the mood for a fabulous sexual encounter. Once things heat up between you, you can hit "stop" on the remote, or leave the film playing for a background of sexy moans and grunts.

You may see something in a video—an interesting sexual position, an activity you've thought about trying, a location or scene that turns you on—that inspires you to try it out with your partner. A video can be a good way to illustrate a specific desire or fantasy, a visual explanation you can give your partner. You can role-play or act out something you see on the screen, adding your own unique flavor rather than copying it exactly. There are also plenty of superb educational adult videos that can teach you new techniques. Porn can also give you some pointers on dirty talk!

Porn can also illustrate and validate your own desires. I once showed a friend a magazine pictorial of two women having sex in a dressing room. "Wow!" she said, "I have Macy's fantasies all the time, but I never knew anyone else did!" After watching a video with porn star Chloe, whose primary orgasmic experience is through penetration rather than clitoral stimulation, a woman told me, "I totally identified with Chloe and how she comes! I've never been that into oral sex or clit stimulation, and my boyfriends are always surprised that I can have an orgasm through intercourse alone. The way that Chloe orgasms is so similar to my own sexual experience. She makes me feel like I'm normal." By seeing ourselves on the page or screen, we can feel assured that our sexual desires, identities, and experiences are shared by others.

One factor that motivated me to produce my video *The Ultimate Guide to Anal Sex for Women* is that people can *learn* from porn. Certainly, there are plenty of outstanding self-help-style instructional videos that are geared toward learning, but people also learn about positions, safer sex, penetration techniques, and plenty more from noninstructional videos.

Until fairly recently, if a couple was interested in introducing porn into their relationship, there weren't a whole lot of

The Best of Classic Porn Performers

- Nina Hartley
- Vanessa del Rio
- Jamie Gillis
- Veronica Hart
- John Holmes
- Richard Pachecho
- Georgina Spelvin
- Marilyn Chambers
- Ginger Lynn

choices. Porn was primarily made by and for men, and it showed that bias; videos contained stereotypical images of women acting out male fantasies with little regard at all for female pleasure. Because the typical porn video was so blatantly male-focused, men were embarrassed to watch it with their female partners, and with good reason. Many women were either offended, disgusted, bored or simply not aroused by the porn that was out there.

But there are some terrific "golden oldies" from the *Boogie Nights* era when porn was shot on film. Before video technology was introduced, porn movies were made much like mainstream movies, and many had substantial budgets. As a result, there are some movies that still stand the test of time, as long as you don't mind the retro 1970s fashion, hairdos, and music. (I like to think of them as historical texts, which makes them charming *and* educational.) Classics like *Behind the Green Door, Insatiable, New Wave Hookers,* and *The Devil in Miss Jones* are still popular rentals at video stores and in mail-order catalogs.

Today, the adult industry is thriving and growing at an unbelievable rate. The market has diversified tremendously, offering consumers an immense variety of products to choose from. There are close to one thousand new titles released each month in many different genres, styles, and formats.[20] If you are interested in sampling what's out there, first you may want to consider what genres appeal to you.

Full-blown features are shot on either film or video and have the ambitions of a mainstream movie with explicit sex added. Within the feature genre, there are realistic dramas, action/adventure movies, historical or period pieces, sci-fi and fantasy creations, and even the occasional comedy. Feature covers usually look like regular movie box covers; some may be sexier, while some show no nudity at all on the front. If you can do without plots and characters and just want to cut to the chase, then all-sex (also called wall-to-wall) and gonzo videos are more your speed; some all-sex videos have a theme that may be all-girl, all-anal, or all-blow-jobs—you can usually tell by the title. If you're looking for the real thing, then amateur or pro-am videos give it to you, with real people, many in their virgin on-screen voyages. To add to the list, there are also sex-instruction videos; independent/alternative videos, BDSM and fetish videos; lesbian, gay, bisexual and transsexual videos; and extremely specialized titles (like women-over-sixty, pregnant-women, or tickling videos). You can read detailed reviews of videos in many adult-store catalogs, on retail video Web sites, and in publications like *Adult Video News* and *Adam Film World*.

Porn for Couples

Luckily, the couples market in porn has grown substantially in the last fifteen years. In 1984, former adult actress Candida Royalle created Femme Productions, a company devoted to producing erotic videos from a woman's point of view. Not feminist per se, and certainly not soft-core, as many assume they are, Royalle's videos are full of realistic characters, interesting story lines, and passionate sex with a focus on women's pleasure. Titles like *The Bridal Shower, One Size Fits All,* and *Eyes of Desire 1* and *2* combine well-crafted stories with seduction, foreplay,

Adult Movies to Watch

Drama: *Artemesia, Bad Habits, Bad Wives, Being with Juli Ashton, Bobby Sox, Cashmere, The Cult, Dinner Party at 6, Every Woman Has a Fantasy 2 and 3, Exstasy, Eyes of Desire 1 and 2, Flashpoint, Heartache, Heart & Soul, Hidden Obsessions, Intimate Expressions, Isis Blue, Justine: Nothing to Hide 2, The Kiss, Looker, Love's Passion, The Masseuse, Models, My Surrender, Red Vibe Diaries, Secret Garden, Sensual Exposure, Shipwreck, Still Insatiable, Torn, West Side, Zazel, The Zone*

Fantasy: *Babylon, Cafe Flesh 1 and 2, Dark Angels, Dark Garden, The Devil in Miss Jones 3 and 4, DreamQuest, Eros, Latex, Les Vampyres, Psychosexuals, Satyr, Search for The Snow Leopard, Seven Deadly Sins, Shock*

Comedy: *Blue Movie, Double Feature!, M: Caught in the Act, One Size Fits All*

Historical/Period: *Apassionata, A Midsummer Night's Cream*

romance, and chemistry between partners. The so-called money shot, where a man ejaculates on a woman's face, breasts, or body, is just one feature of traditional adult videos that leaves some women feeling exploited or turned off. Notably, Femme videos are some of the only videos that portray "internal" cum shots.

It took about a decade, but finally some of the biggest and brightest adult-video companies have caught up with Candida Royalle and are producing high-quality porn videos marketed for couples. The formula of this new breed of porn is based on a simplistic model of Mars and Venus. Show enough sucking and fucking to appeal to the average guy (after all, he's still the easiest target). Soften said activities with characters, dialogue, and production values, so these same guys won't be embarrassed to watch it with their wives. The fact that women may also get off

Standout Adult Directors

Brad Armstrong	Antonio Passolini
Juli Ashton	Candida Royalle
Andrew Blake	Ren Savant
Toni English	Paul Thomas
Veronica Hart	Michael Zen
Michael Ninn	

is a bonus. In some cases, with all the emphasis on high production values, the actual sex scenes of these couples features lose the heat and passion of raunchier films. But I am thrilled nonetheless that finally the industry is acknowledging women as consumers of porn, and making products that they can not only stomach but might even enjoy.

Porn for couples includes big-budget features shot on film or video with exotic locations or unique settings. They've got scripts that actually make sense, well-drawn characters, solid acting, and production values that strive to match those of Hollywood. Some even have elaborate concepts or costumes and special effects. The idea is to create a movie like a big blockbuster and instead of R-rated, make it X-rated. One aspect of mainstream porn that may be less than desirable for women is the way many female performers look: perfectly skinny bodies, large fake breasts, and the California Girl/Miss America idea of "beautiful." This cookie-cutter Barbie look still rules, but the tide is turning, and you can find natural-looking women in the business more today than ever before. Now, all this time, effort, and money doesn't necessarily guarantee a great porn flick, but there are some exceptional production companies, directors, and performers worth watching.

If your taste is much softer, and you prefer the implication of sex rather than explicit close-ups of penetration and genitals, your best bet is cable and pay-per-view television channels like Playboy and Spice, which broadcast soft-core versions of adult features; you can also rent installments of the wildly popular cable series *Red Shoe Diaries*.

Adult Stars to Watch

Within the feature genre, there is a new generation of adult performers who have a wonderful combination of qualities. They can give strong acting turns *and* incredible sexual performances. They seem to truly love their work, and their enthusiasm and passion comes through clearly on-screen, especially female performers who have explosive, authentic orgasms. In some but not all cases, many of this next generation have gloriously natural bodies unenhanced by breast implants or other plastic surgery. Some of these stars to watch (along with a few of their film credits) are:

- Shanna McCullough (*Bobby Sox, Looker*)
- James Bonn (*Models, Chloe, Search for the Snow Leopard*)
- Chloe (*The Masseuse 3, Chloe, Misspelled, Club Hades*)
- Jeanna Fine (*Cafe Flesh 2, My Surrender*)
- Sarah-Jane Hamilton (*Pretending, Generally Horny Hospital*)
- Tyffany Million (*Dirty Little Mind, Mind Games*)
- Sean Michaels (*Dinner Party at 6, Sean Michaels Rocks That Ass*)
- Missy (*Eros, One Size Fits All, Heartache*)
- Stephanie Swift (*The Awakening, Miscreants, Shipwreck*)
- Inari Vachs (*The Awakening, Three, Trigger*)

The representation of people of color in mainstream pornography can be pretty dismal, although the company Video Team has a line called Afro-Centric devoted to African-American erotica. In addition, African-American actors Sean

Michaels and Mr. Marcus have directed their own series. Along with Michaels and Marcus, there are several talented actors of color who appear in mainstream videos, among them: Asia Carrera, Stephanie Swift, Heather Hunter, Kobe Tai, Midori, Dee, Tia Bella, Lexington Steele, and Jake Steed.

Just Show Me the Sex

Some porn companies have an entirely different approach to video: ditch the scripts and plots and concentrate on the sex, even if it means some amateurish production values. All-sex videos, also called "wall-to-wall," are down and dirty, sometimes outrageous, and very often have plenty of sexual energy. The theory behind these is that if you don't require actors to memorize lines, act, ride horses, have elaborate costumes or accents, they can concentrate on what they do best: fuck. Some all sex videos are shot *Real World*–style, where the camera (and the person behind it) is acknowledged as part of the storytelling. In this subgenre known as "gonzo," spontaneity, realness, and hot, raw sex are emphasized over stylized plots, sets, and other elements of big-budget productions.

Before the *Survivor–The Real World–Temptation Island* reality-television craze, the adult industry was capitalizing on sexual reality with amateur (sometimes called "pro-am") porn. If you like to see real people who aren't porn stars and have no scripts, or have a look at a nonpro's first fuck on video, you may like this homemade version of adult videos, with titles like *Video Virgins, Filthy First Timers,* and *Totally Amateur.* Watching amateur porn, you have to take the truly spontaneous and sexy moments with the more awkward—his struggle to undo her bra, the weird faces she makes when he licks her pussy, the way his dick slips out of her in a certain position.

Just like on television, there is a danger to realism: it can be boring. Capturing people fucking on film doesn't necessarily make stimulating porn. Sex itself isn't always sexy: it can be

Gonzo Standouts

- John Leslie: Actor-director Leslie's series *The Voyeur* typifies the gonzo style and features uninhibited performers (many of them European), wildly orgasmic encounters, and lots of anal sex.

- Seymore Butts Home Movies: The highlight of actor-director and gonzo master Seymore Butts's line is the performances of the beautiful, anal-sex-loving, ejaculating starlet Alisha Klass (check her out in *Tushy Con Carne* and *Tushy Tampa Fest*).

- *Shane's World:* A blond, bubbly California girl, Shane was a young porn star who conceived and directed her own gonzo series called *Shane's World,* which is full of real female orgasms, giggling and high jinks, fresh talent, newcomers, impromptu how-to demos, and safer sex.

- Chloe: Award-winning actress Chloe has also begun directing some highly entertaining, sexy gonzo movies, including *Chloe's What Makes You Cum?, I Came, Did You?,* and *Chloe's Catalina Cum-Ons.*

clumsy, and it's not always as well paced as a finely directed feature. Actual erotic moments can also lack drama and intensity—have you seen the Tonya Harding wedding-night video? Sex can be a very individual, internal experience that's hard to capture if people don't externalize their feelings. I admit it's interesting to watch real unguarded, unjaded people go at it sometimes, and certainly watching a woman have a real orgasm is way more fun than watching her fake one. Amateur porn is usually hit or miss, but some of the most consistently entertaining series are *Homegrown Video, Up and Cummers,* and *Dirty Debutantes* (if you can stomach their star and director, Ed Powers).

Other Porn Genres

In addition to features, gonzo, and amateur, here are some other genres which may appeal to couples:

How-To/Instructional: To learn something while you're getting off, look for Nina Hartley's How-To series, masturbation guru Betty Dodson's educational tapes, as well as Deborah Sundahl's *How to Female Ejaculate* and *Tantric Journey to Female Orgasm.* Much more traditional and less uninhibited is the Sinclair Intimacy Institute's Better Sex Video Series.

Girl/Girl: Mainstream titles which feature girls doing girls for a primarily male audience. They tend to focus on women with long fingernails (which no real lesbian would be caught dead with) touching tongue-to-tongue (think *Playboy* pictorials). They aren't usually portrayed as lesbians, and they don't always emphasize women getting off.

Lesbian: Porn produced by lesbians and starring lesbians (usually amateurs) is a rarity, except for videos from companies such as Fatale Video, S.I.R. Video, and Maria Beatty's Bleu Productions.

Gay: Perhaps surprisingly, some women—both straight and lesbian—really enjoy gay male porn. Straight women often watch gay male porn for the actors, because the truth is that gay porn actors are a dozen times better looking, better endowed, more well-groomed, -oiled and -muscled than most guys in straight porn. If women can get over the fact that the guys are fucking each other and there are no chicks in sight, they're in for some handsome eye candy and raw, no-holds-barred sexual energy.

Bisexual: Sadly, when it comes to bisexual porn, worthwhile titles are few and far between. One reason is that the industries are so divided that no one is permitted to cross over or act in both gay and straight porn without being ostracized by both sides. As a result, there aren't enough actors who'll do bi porn and producers who care enough to focus on it. But you'll always be able to spot the bisexual vids at the store by their hilarious, revealing titles: *The Hills Have Bis, Bi Bi Love, Remembering Times Gone Bi, Every Switch Way* . . . You get the picture.

BDSM: Because of local obscenity standards, mainstream S/M videos rarely combine S/M with sex. Dubbed the "Master of Fetish Erotica," director-actor Ernest Greene has made some of the finest S/M and fetish porn ever created, with attractive and enthusiastic performers, spectacular fetish clothing and equipment, and accurate representations of kinky fantasies (Greene really knows his stuff). Bizarre Video also produces some of the most diverse BDSM/fetish porn in the industry, from bondage and master/slave play to enemas to golden showers.

While pornography is often made and marketed toward specific audiences, that shouldn't make you think that if you are straight, you should only watch and enjoy straight porn. The world of porn is often black and white, with its hard and fast categories like "gay," "S/M," or "for men." These labels assume a direct correspondence between a user's identity and her or his tastes in smut. Well, the fact of the matter is that straight men do not look at only straight erotic magazines, lesbians do not only watch lesbian videos, and women do not only read women's erotica. Never underestimate the possibility that our libidos don't always conveniently match up with our sexual identities; they can be a lot more perverse than we may think. That's another wonderful feature of porn—you have the opportunity to witness sexual people and activities entirely outside of your own experience. The thing about porn is that it's very individual, tastes vary, and you cannot always anticipate what will turn you or your partner on and what might not do the trick whatsoever!

Femme and Beyond

Femme Productions definitely paved the way for a growing list of movies for those girls who like a little conversation with their cock. Just doing away with that money shot was progress. Women have a very different relationship to visual pornography than men, and female fans are a lot more complicated—some want it nasty, some want it sweet, and plenty want it both ways!

In fact, even though I criticized it, I admit there are some women who *like* to watch the infamous semen-on-the-face image. I know women who do; there are just fewer of them than the men who love it. And that's okay. Just because the adult industry calls a video "couples-oriented" and says this is what you should like doesn't mean you have to like it! Money shot or no money shot, hardcore gonzo or well-scripted feature, it's all up to you and your partner. If you are a woman who enjoys watching S/M videos with women being dominated by men, don't feel bad or guilty about it. It doesn't necessarily mean you want to be dominated or want other women to be in real life. It's just fantasy.

Some of the more savvy video stores and catalogs now have a "couples" section to help point you in the right direction. If that is not the case, and you don't feel comfortable asking friends or video store employees for recommendations, you can pick up an industry magazine like *Adult Video News* or a comprehensive book like *The Couple's Guide to the Best Erotic Videos* for detailed reviews. You can watch several different kinds of videos to see what genres, companies, directors, performers, and styles appeal to you. Discuss your likes and dislikes with your partner. Sample titles until you find what turns you on. Grab the remote, and let the fun begin.

Why do some porn videos show condom use and others don't?

The depiction of safer sex in adult film has been a complex and controversial issue since HIV and AIDS have become a growing concern in America. For a long time, the entire straight mainstream industry did not represent condom use or safer sex practices in any of its films. In the 1990s, when several prominent performers were diagnosed with HIV, and it was determined that at least some of them had become infected from a co-worker on the set of a film, the industry finally woke up. Several individual performers as well as entire production companies proclaimed themselves "condom only"—using condoms for each and every penetrative scene in a movie. Other producers decided to be condom-optional or condom-free, arguing that people want to see fantasies in porn, not the reality of latex barriers for protection, or that it is up to the individual performers to decide. Today, it remains a murky, unresolved issue. If you want to see 100 percent condom use in your videos, look for movies by VCA, Vivid, Wicked Pictures, and Video Team (movies shot in the U.S. only).[21]

BEYOND WHIPS AND CHAINS

Exploring BDSM

Have you ever imagined being tied up by your lover? Does the thought of being forced to do something turn you on? Would spanking your boyfriend arouse you? Do you like the idea of surrendering control to someone dominant? Perhaps in your fantasies, you are slowly dripping hot wax on your girlfriend's breasts. Or you are blindfolding your husband and teasing him. Maybe you want your nipples pinched harder and for longer than most people. Or the sensation of being whipped makes you feel high. If any of these activities sound exciting or inspiring, then welcome to the wonderful world of BDSM.

Definitions

BDSM is an umbrella term that encompasses a range of activities, including one or more of the following: physical dominance and submission, psychological dominance and submission, bondage, and pain. BDSM always involves an exchange of power between two people that is erotic to both of them, although not necessarily specifically sexual. BDSM is an intimate journey that people take together, a journey that allows them to explore the boundaries of pain and pleasure, the limits of their own minds and bodies, and even altered states of consciousness. What does BDSM stand for? It's a clever combination of three distinct but related terms: B&D, D&S, and S/M. Bondage and discipline ("B&D") is just what it sounds like—restraining someone in a variety of different ways, and punishing them or keeping them in line, either physically or verbally (or both). If tying someone up appeals to you, then you're into bondage. Ever get the urge to play a strict governess, an exacting teacher, or a cruel drill sergeant? Then you like discipline. Put 'em together, and you're doing B&D.

Dominance and submission ("D&S") is a dynamic in which one person is dominant and the other is submissive. The focus of D&S is on the way partners relate to one another; the dominant is clearly in control, and the submissive gives in to his or her wishes. Of course, D&S may be combined with B&D or S/M, but it doesn't have to be. Submissives give themselves completely over to their dominants; a submissive serves and pleases a dominant, whose needs and wishes come first. If you're bossy, like to make the rules and run the show, then you've got the makings of a dominant; on the other hand, if you're a pleaser, like to follow someone else's lead, or get pleasure from doing things for other people, there just might be a submissive hiding inside you. Master-and-slave play is a typical example of a D&S relationship.

Sadism and masochism, or sadomasochism (S/M), is the exploration of sensations that flirt with the boundary between pleasure and pain. Sadists enjoy inflicting pain, discomfort, punishment, or cruelty upon others, and masochists enjoy being on the receiving end. Examples of sadomasochistic activities include: flogging, caning, sensory deprivation, nipple clamps, and hot wax, which may be combined with different types of psychological play.

People who are unfamiliar with S/M often cannot understand how pain can be erotic, pleasurable, and even desirable.

We usually associate pain with physical discomfort and suffering. Sex is supposed to be about feeling good, and what feels good about pain? Well, in actuality, pain can be extremely pleasurable for some people. For one thing, there is a very fine distinction between pleasure and pain, and many people like to explore sensations that test that line, as well as their endurance, strength, and resilience. Also, when the body experiences pain, it releases endorphins and other chemicals that attempt to inhibit the pain; these hormones may cause you to feel aroused, euphoric, or high. S/M play may also have an intense emotional component, in which someone has the opportunity to test boundaries and explore fantasies and even fears. Role-playing can be a chance to investigate erotically charged power dynamics. Some S/M practitioners describe their experiences as deeply spiritual. When they play, they can achieve different states of consciousness as well as connect with their own bodies and their lovers.

BDSM experiences are outside the "norm" of sexual practices, but that doesn't mean that BDSM is not normal—there is a difference. Cultural and societal norms shift and change, and BDSM practices are more accepted by mainstream institutions than ever before. Psychiatry took S/M off its list of mental disorders back in the eighties, and a recent *Psychology Today* article touted: "Such desires are increasingly being considered normal, even healthy, as experts begin to recognize their potential psychological value. . . . S&M, they are beginning to understand, offers a release of sexual and emotional energy that some people cannot get from traditional sex."[22] I have learned from working at a sex-toy store and teaching workshops that a large percentage of the general public has experimented at least once with some form of BDSM, whether it's being tied up, delivering a spanking, or slipping a blindfold on a lover.

People often describe BDSM with the term "play," as in, "I'd love to play with her" or "We played together at the conference in Baltimore." Sometimes play can be light and fun, but don't let the word fool you: play can also be complex, serious, and very profound. I use the term "play" simply to describe doing BDSM. While we are on the subject of terminology, a "scene" is when two people come together to do BDSM play.

Are You a Top, a Bottom, or a Switch?

BDSM begins when you decide which role you'd like to embody for a specific scene. Basically, you need to ask yourself this question: do you want to be dishing it out or taking it? If you want to be dishing it out, then you're a top, and if you want to take it, you're a bottom. If you think you might like to do both, then you may be a switch.

There are lots of different kinds of tops. In general, tops like to be in charge, run the show, and do things to someone else (namely the bottom). A top is usually the aggressor and initiator, and definitely takes a more active role than the bottom. In B&D, tops are the ones who administer discipline and punishment. In D&S, the top is the dominant, and in S/M, the top is the sadist or has a sadistic streak. If you relate and connect to these characteristics, enjoy being in control and having power, become aroused at the idea of inflicting pain or discomfort, or revel in the thought of someone serving your needs and desires, then you very well may be a top.

What makes a good top? Almost nothing can match years of experience at negotiating and creating scenes and practicing BDSM skills. A top who is exceptionally talented at a particular activity is wonderful, and someone who genuinely enjoys doing what he or she is doing is even better. Some of the most sought-after tops in the BDSM scene are not the most attractive, well dressed, or flashy. They are caring, sensitive, intuitive people; they have a gift for assessing a bottom's needs and meeting them, figuring out a bottom's boundaries and buttons and then pushing them. I also appreciate a creative top, one who can challenge me, catch me off guard, maybe even scare me when it is appropriate. What qualifies as a good top also really depends on the bottom: some want a very strict top, where others appreciate someone who won't be a hard-ass all the time. Some people want a very dominant top who overpowers and commands them, while others are satisfied with someone willing to simply take the lead. There are also plenty of people who appreciate a top who has a flair for the dramatic. I can always spot a theater major at the dungeon: she's usually got a good sense of pacing, a quick tongue, and a well-planned erotic drama. No matter what their style or specific skills, when someone obviously derives pleasure from being a top, their enjoyment can be infectious.

Like tops, bottoms can be a diverse and unique bunch of people. Many bottoms enjoy having things done *to* them, whether that means being tied up, being beaten, or being dominated. Some bottoms are passive, and others are not. Bottoms like to be the object of the top's affection, desire, and, perhaps, cruelty or discipline. They prefer to give up control, surrender to another person, follow someone else's orders. Some bottoms are submissive, others are masochistic, and many are a wonderful combination of both. If you crave attention, discipline, or pain or have the desire to serve someone else, you've got the makings of a bottom.

First and foremost, in order to be a good bottom, you need to know what you want and be able to express your desires to your partner. Bottoms who know their bodies and their physical and emotional needs and limits are appreciated by tops; this knowledge comes with experience. The more BDSM play you do, the better you are at figuring out what you like and what you don't. When a bottom can go the distance—take an intense flogging, give perfect service, push herself to go beyond one of her limits—a top is in heaven. What makes a good bottom can be quite subjective, depending on individual tastes: some people want a bottom to be passive, submissive, and unquestioning, bowing to authority completely. Others appreciate a masochist who gets off on pain or a bottom who is very service-oriented, deriving pleasure simply from doing things for a top. Everyone appreciates a responsive bottom—it's no fun to do something to someone who doesn't react at all!

Perhaps all this talk of giving and taking has you thinking that you'd actually like to do both. Well, then, you are a switch. Contrary to some popular thinking, switches are not just wishy-washy folks who can't make up their minds. Switches are people who like to see things from both sides and take different positions depending on the particular situation. You may start out wanting to experience different aspects of BDSM from both ends, doling it out and taking it, then find you come to see you really do fit into one or the other. But don't feel like you have to choose right away or identify yourself to the world at large. Focus on what you want rather than what label applies to you.

The important thing to remember is that these roles do not need to be set in stone. You are absolutely free to change your mind or change your position depending on your mood, the person you're with, or what you'd like to get from a BDSM experience. You can be a spanking top, a bondage bottom, and a sensory-deprivation switch. But before you do anything, you need to negotiate with your partner and learn how to make a BDSM scene safe, sane, and consensual.

Negotiation

Because BDSM encompasses so many different practices, people who do BDSM like to talk with their partners first about their likes and dislikes. This is one of the very best things that BDSM has taught me: how to determine what you want, clearly tell someone, and then get that person to do it to you! I am a big fan of being very direct, as I hope you know by now. A good way to begin negotiating with your partner is to write three lists for each other. I apologize in advance if this sounds way too Martha Stewart organized, but we're playing with some rough stuff here, and it's all about boundaries. What are your boundaries and what are your partner's? Make a "Yes List" of things you'd like to do. Write a "No List" of activities you absolutely don't want to do. Create a "Maybe List" and include anything you may consider doing under the right circumstances. There may also be details or limits within these lists. For example: yes to flogging—but only light to medium. Or: no to cutting—you can tease or threaten me with knives, just don't actually use them on me! Later in this chapter, I will discuss various BDSM practices to give you some ideas about what to put on your lists.

In addition to BDSM activities, you need to determine whether you also want to incorporate sexual play into your scene. Plenty of people who do BDSM get off on it without ever having their genitals touched or engaging in sex. So, you may want to decide that you want to do BDSM without any sex at all. Or, you may say "yes" to sex, with some rules, like, "If you're going to tie me up, I will feel especially vulnerable, so no anal penetration please."

One of the tenets of BDSM that practitioners are very serious about is the concept that all BDSM play should be "safe, sane, and consensual." Safe: everyone involved in the BDSM exchange must be safe from physical harm, including the transmission of disease. Sane: partners should communicate with each other, be emotionally stable, and respect each other's physical and emotional boundaries. Consensual: each person must give his or her consent to what happens. Here are some more tips about how to go about making BDSM play safe, sane, and consensual for you.

Here are some activities you may want to include on your "Yes," "No," and "Maybe" lists:

biting	hoods
blindfolds	hot wax play
bondage	humiliation
caning	paddling
clamps, nipple	pinching
clamps, other	role playing
collar and leash	shaving
discipline	slapping
flogging	spanking
gags	scratching

Making BDSM Play Safe

In order to insure the physical and emotional safety of your partner, it's important to know as much as you can about him or her. A person's medical history must be taken into consideration before you decide what kinds of things you are going to do together. For example, does your partner have a heart condition, high blood pressure, hypoglycemia, asthma, allergies, or a history of fainting? Is she taking any medication that may affect her physical or emotional state? Are there areas of his body that were previously injured and should be avoided? Does she have sensitive spots with which you need to take extra care? This is all good information to have before you start swinging a whip someone's way or doing anything else, really. If you are going to add sex to the mix, you also want to set down some guidelines for safer sex practices.

When it comes to most BDSM practices, you cannot simply pick up a candle and start dripping. First, you need to learn how to do whatever it is you want correctly and safely, then you need to practice—preferably on an inanimate object rather than your bottom—before actually doing it. So, how do you learn how to do BDSM? There are dozens of books on the subject, both general overviews (like *SM 101* and *Screw the Roses, Send Me the Thorns*) and books with very specific topics (like *The Erotic Bondage Handbook* and *The Compleat Spanker*). There are also a few videos, including Frank and Ona Zee's introductory series called *Learning the Ropes*. Find out if there is a local BDSM support group or organization in your community where you can meet other kinky people. You may want to go to a play party or a local S/M club, where you can see people engaged in BDSM. If you see something you'd like to know more about, don't interrupt anyone's scene, but wait until they are finished and politely ask some questions. Attending BDSM workshops and demonstrations is another great way to learn safe techniques from skilled and experienced BDSM practitioners. I will also offer tips on a select group of practices later in this chapter.

Once you have studied up and practiced, the first time that you try something out, start small. Do not try to do too much too soon: a well-executed spanking is much more appreciated than an overly ambitious scene of a sloppy caning, a rushed paddling, and a scattered flogging. Go slow. Use your common sense and trust your instincts. Listen to the verbal and nonverbal cues of your bottom. Take your time.

Keeping BDSM Play Sane

Because BDSM can be very intense, it's important that both partners come to it with, well, clear heads. If you are feeling particularly unstable, stressed out, or vulnerable for any reason, it's probably best to postpone your scene until you feel emotionally ready. In addition to discussing physical safety, you want to make sure that you and your partner are emotionally safe. Ask if there are any particular words, actions, or scenarios that may trigger someone in a negative way; for example, I know a woman who suffered physical abuse as a child. As an adult, she likes to be spanked with a variety of implements *except* wooden spoons. Many men do not want to be forced into a feminine role or made to cross-dress. For some people, yelling cannot be part of a discipline scene. The idea is for both people to approach each other with respect and responsibility. Realize that setting these limits and discussing them beforehand still may not prevent someone from having an emotional response during a scene: be prepared so that if something comes up, you will be there to support your partner.

Since we are talking about keeping your scene sane, you may also want to consider how you feel about alcohol and drugs combined with BDSM. I never use drugs or alcohol if I am going to do a scene with someone, and I ask that my partners refrain from them as well. Drugs and alcohol impair your judgment and your communication skills, lessen your inhibitions, and decrease your ability to execute physical tasks skillfully. If you are under the influence of drugs or alcohol, you may be more inclined to cross a boundary that you wouldn't if you were sober. Your senses are also impaired, and your pain tolerance will be off kilter. You could hurt someone or yourself. For all these reasons, they just aren't a good match for safe and sane BDSM.

Consensual BDSM

Sharing your lists of likes and dislikes and talking to each other before you play helps both people give their consent to the activities you are going to embark on together. As you review your lists, ask your partner to elaborate about a specific activity and what they like or don't like about it. This can give you great insight into their desires and overall approach to the scene. Before you begin, you should also negotiate with your bottom about marking his or her body, since many BDSM activities, like a light caning or a heavy flogging, can leave marks on the skin.

You should also both agree to use a safeword during a scene. A safeword is a word—usually one that you wouldn't normally utter during a scene—that you and your partner choose. Your safeword is your safety net. If you don't like something that's happening or you want the scene to stop right away, use your safeword. So, why don't you just say "Stop"? Well, in some cases, part of the turn-on for people is to be made to do something "against their will." So, saying "stop" or "no" or "please don't" is part of the dialogue of the scene. A safeword shouldn't be one of these words or phrases, it should be something altogether different.

Safewords are one way to help insure that everyone feels secure in the scene. Sometimes, it can be quite challenging to communicate with your partner during a scene, especially if you are role-playing and taking your top or bottom status very seriously. In those cases, things you might normally say to each other during sex—"How does that feel, honey? Am I hurting you?" or "Go slower, I don't like it so fast; okay, I'm ready for more now"—might not work in a BDSM context. That kind of banter could throw off the dynamic completely. That's why communication and negotiation prior to the scene is so crucial. As a top, you need to be creative in communicating with your bottom. Find interesting ways to let the bottom have his or her say, while still maintaining the notion that you are the one in control. One way to do this is to tell the bottom that she or he needs to ask (or maybe beg) for the next cane stroke, another hit from the paddle, or whatever it is you are doing. That way, when the bottom asks, you know he or she is ready for it—it also adds to the erotic dynamic between you. If you aren't sure if you are pacing something correctly, you may want to ask the bottom; you can keep questions simple without breaking out of your roles.

After your scene is over, it's a good idea to have an informal debriefing session, just to check in with your partner and see how the scene was for him or her. Doing BDSM with someone can be extremely intense. People can have different reactions to it and might need to talk afterward. You should be ready to listen and reassure. The processing of a scene may last for several days or into the next week, so be prepared for that.

Creating a Scene

Think of a BDSM scene as your own private drama, in which you and your partner are the writers, directors, producers, and stars. The elements of a good scene are similar to those of a piece of theater: you need interesting characters, smart dialogue, a strong setting, cool costumes and props, and a plot (or at least a theme or chain of events). Many people often approach a BDSM scene as a ritual in which each moment is symbolic of the connection two partners create.

Ideally, you will be able to explore BDSM in the comfort and privacy of your own home, but that may not be feasible. Do you live in an apartment building with very thin walls? Do you have roommates who may be freaked out if they hear you playing? Do you have children who will be within earshot? If you think you might make some out-of-the-ordinary noises, like skin being smacked, beating sounds, or lots of moaning and shouting, that may affect where your scenes take place. If you cannot play where you live, you have several options. Perhaps you can ask another kinky friend to use his or her place. You could go to a local hotel and request a room with the most privacy (tell them you're going to rehearse a performance art piece and don't want to disturb other guests). If you would enjoy playing in public, perhaps you can attend an S/M club or a play party. For special occasions, local dungeons (where clients have sessions with professional dominatrices) often rent rooms by the hour.

Wherever you choose to play, it is important to create a space that is both safe and functional for your scene. If you're in your own home, it may be nice to do away with the distractions of everyday life: turn the phone's ringer off, change the lighting, cover the computer. Sometimes it is easier for people to slip into their role if their space doesn't remind them of their job, family, and day-to-day stresses. Make sure you have everything you need at hand—sex toys, condoms, lube, safer sex supplies, that perfect CD in the stereo. Nothing kills a mood like running out of the room and rummaging around for something.

If you decide you are a top or you're going to be one for the evening, you have taken on the planning role of the scene: you need to figure out what you're going to do and how you're gonna do it. You should decide what specific role you'd like to play—the dominant, the sadist, the disciplinarian, a combination of several, or another role altogether. What would you like to be called—Mistress, Master, Sir, Ma'am, Miss, Goddess, something else? Who shall your bottom be—slave, boy, girl?

Your chosen characters will, of course, depend on your chosen scene, what it revolves around, what its theme is. Will it be the Mistress and her slave, the King and his servant, the Governess and a naughty boy? Will there be an after-school detention with spanking by ruler or a fraternity hazing scene with blindfolds and paddling? Will it be simply top and bottom in a prolonged caning scene or two switches coating each other with hot wax?

Planning is wonderful, but as the scene goes on, make sure that you are flexible. Even if you mapped out the perfect sequence of spanking, bondage, and hot wax, be able to go with the flow if you sense that something isn't working or both of you want to go in a different direction. Don't be afraid to change the plot midway through a scene; in most cases, the bottom will never know the difference because she or he will be having such a great time. Especially when you are starting out, don't set your expectations too high; remember you are still figuring things out and there are sure to be a few bumps along the way. When the scene is over, most people need some care afterward, such as some cuddling, support, gentle stroking, and reassurance; no matter what you do, it's important to be fully present for each other, since you both just underwent an intense experience together.

So . . . Let's Play!

There are literally dozens of practices which fall under the heading of BDSM, too many to name in just one chapter. Plus, a detailed description and discussion of each practice is impossible to do in only one chapter. In reality, you need an entire book to do justice to the depth and breadth of BDSM. Here, I offer you a sampling of some of the most popular BDSM practices. These activities are pleasurable on their own, and can of course be combined within one scene. I want to emphasize that these are some of the basics—think S/M 101. There are plenty of other crazy things for you to do, but let's start simple, shall we?

Bondage

Bondage is the physical restraint of someone's body (or a part of his or her body) by a variety of different means. When people are in bondage, they often feel physically vulnerable to the person who tied them up. Putting someone into bondage automatically gives you the upper hand, since a bottom will likely feel at the mercy of the top. Bondage is a wonderful way to give up control, and for some bottoms, it's a perfect way to get into a submissive role. All of these feelings can be highly erotic to people who enjoy bondage. Bondage tops take pleasure in restraining their bottoms, overpowering them, even "trapping" them. If you have ever held your partner's wrists down to the bed, you are practicing a basic form of bondage.

You don't necessarily have to invest in elaborate equipment to put someone in bondage. You can use common items you have around the house to tie a bottom's wrists or ankles together, including scarves, neckties, belts, robe ties, very thick ribbon, nylon, or even a dog leash (not the chain variety). However—and this may come as bad news to you—if you've got those ubiquitous metal handcuffs, you need to retire them. Though they are sold as adult novelties and are seen in bedrooms all over the country, they really are not safe to use to restrain someone. Most handcuffs do not have a working safety latch to keep them from closing too tightly around the wrist; they can restrict circulation, cut into wrists, and do serious damage to someone. Keep the handcuffs around as props, but don't actually use them! Similarly, beginners should avoid using tape of any kind as well as restraints made of metal or wire; they are not safe if you don't have experience with them.

If you want to spend some money to tie up your lover, you can purchase a whole range of wrist and ankle restraints at leather, S/M, and sex-toy stores (see illustration 9). Made of nylon, leather, or rubber, many restraints are lined with a soft material to make them more comfortable. Restraints are an easy way to put someone in bondage, since you simply slip them around the wrists and ankles, then attach them together (with a panic snap or clip, sold with restraints or at any hardware store). Once the ankles or wrists are joined together, you can also attach the restraints to bed posts, a futon frame, a chair, or some other sturdy piece of furniture.

If you'd like to use rope for bondage, it's important to use rope that is soft and strong. Cotton rope is fairly soft, and you can wash it a few times to make it even softer. Make sure, however, that it's pure cotton rope (a good source is a magician's-supply store), since a lot of so-called cotton rope (like clothesline rope) is actually cotton over plastic tubing, which isn't good for bondage. Nylon rope is also soft and good for

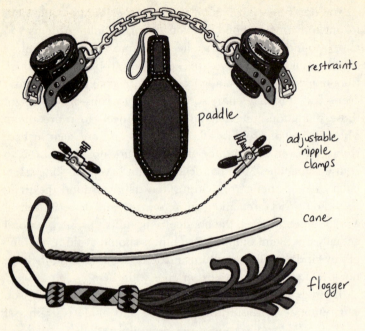

restraints

paddle

adjustable nipple clamps

cane

flogger

FIG. 9 BDSM TOYS

bondage, although it can be too silky to hold a knot. Strong and washable, nylon climbing rope and webbing are great for bondage.

Whether you use rope or another material, keep the knots simple and easy to untie. Do not tie knots too tightly—you don't want to cut off the bottom's circulation. If you need to brush up on tying techniques, there are plenty of books (geared for sailors and other outdoor sportsmen) that explain how to tie easy knots. Make sure that the bottom is in a position that will not put any undue strain on the body. For example, if you tie someone spread-eagle to a bed, don't spread their arms or legs too far apart. You never want bondage to put excess strain on parts of the body; the bottom won't be able to be in that bondage for very long. Better to make your captive more comfortable, so she or he can stay tied up for as long as you want!

Bondage Tricks

- *Test the Waters:* If your partner isn't sure how she will feel being tied up, give her a harmless introduction by holding her wrists together above her head with your own hands. See how she responds before you whip out the restraints.

- *Invisible Bondage:* One way to test your partner's submission is to instruct him to keep his hands behind his back or above his head *without* tying him up. Force him to stay in that position as if he were bound. One false move, and he gets another stroke of the cane. You can continue to punish or reward him depending on how well he does.

- *Be Creative:* You don't always need to tie someone's hands above the head. Tie her wrists together with one hand on top of the other. Then, tie her hands between her legs, forcing her to touch herself whenever her body moves.

- *Tease Your Bottom:* Tie your partner up, then tease him mercilessly. Straddle him with your naked body, rub his cock on your pussy, wave your breasts in his face, show him your ass. Make sure to keep yourself just out of reach, and he'll be begging for you in no time!

- *Give Her Something to Think About:* Using about twelve feet of rope, tie it just above her hipbones several times, then run it between her butt cheeks and between her labia. If you're feeling ambitious, tie a knot right against her clitoris. Continue on with the scene, making sure she has plenty of opportunity to feel the rope move between her legs.

If you are more ambitious, and would like to learn to create full-body bondage or a specialized apparatus like a rope bondage harness, then your best source for learning may be a workshop where you can see three-dimensional demonstrations. There are a few informative videos on the subject, including: *Learning the Ropes* volumes 1 and 4 and *Fetish FAQ 1: Bondage. Jay Wiseman's Erotic Bondage Handbook* is the most comprehensive book on bondage and has excellent detailed techniques and illustrations.

One of the most critical factors in bondage is to keep the bottom restrained, yet not seriously physically uncomfortable. The bound partner can be a little uncomfortable but should never be in agony. You always want to make sure that the bondage is fairly easy for you to get the person out of. It sounds like a contradiction, but the truth is that if the bottom suddenly feels ill, claustrophobic, or on the verge of a panic attack, you want to be able to get them out of whatever they are in with relative speed. If you are using rope, that may mean cutting them out of the bondage, so keep a pair of good scissors nearby. Whatever is restraining them should be comfortable against the skin and joints without rubbing, chafing, or cutting into anything. Bondage should never cut off the circulation at any point; if the bottom feels pins and needles or the skin turns blue, you need to undo the bondage right away.

Collars

The collar is an important symbol among BDSM folks. I include it in the bondage section because, to me, a collar around the neck is a more subtle, emotional form of bondage. It may signify ownership, submission, subservience, surrender, and a whole range of other power dynamics. When my lover puts a collar around my neck, it helps me to give up control and become more passive and submissive. Putting a collar on someone is also a great way to begin a scene, to transition from your real personalities into the roles you've chosen. You can find collars designed for people in leather, S/M, and sex-toy stores, but you may also find less expensive ones big enough for humans at pet stores. A collar should be snug around the neck, but never tight, choking, or cutting off circulation. You can also attach a leash to the front of a collar or tie someone's already bound wrists to his or her collar. While gentle tugging at a collar can be a turn-on, never yank a collar, as you can give someone whiplash.

Sensory Deprivation

Depriving someone of one or more of their senses can be an incredible exchange of power. When you take away one sense, the others are greatly heightened. A person who is blindfolded, for example, can concentrate on what's being done to his or her body without any visual distractions, and the physical sensations usually feel more intense as a result. Sensory deprivation can help a bottom focus more on a particular activity like a flogging, caning, or the simple act of dragging your fingernails across the skin. Taking away a bottom's ability to see is also an exercise of control over him or her. Because we process so much critical information through sight, a blindfold or hood can also be used to intimidate, frighten, or trick someone with complex psychological play. One of the very first times that I was put in a hood, the top told me that she was taking me to the local pizza parlor. We drove around for a while, and when she took me out of the car and indoors, she said something like, "Don't worry, she's okay," as if to a concerned onlooker. I truly believed we were in the pizza place, when we were actually just in her apartment!

Some elements of sensory deprivation include blindfolds, gags, and hoods. You can purchase different types of blindfolds at leather, S/M, and sex-toy stores, or you can use sleep masks,

Sensory Deprivation Tricks

- *Taste This:* Don't have a gag handy? Strip your lover down, take off her underwear, and shove it in her mouth. She may feel naughty or shameful, and you'll definitely catch her off guard.

- *Let Your Mouth Wander:* Once he's blindfolded and not looking you straight in the eyes, take the opportunity to practice talking dirty to him. It may be easier for you to find your inner dominatrix, feel less inhibited, and say things you've always wanted to say. Here's your chance to be strict, cruel, or intimidating.

- *Electrify the Senses:* Experiment with the softness of a piece of fur, the chill of an ice cube, the feel of nails dragging on skin, the sharpness of a cold metal implement. All these different sensations will feel twice as intense to a bottom wearing a blindfold or a hood.

- *Tell a Story:* A blindfolded and gagged bottom is a captive audience, so spin a tale about what turns you on, or what you're going to do next, or a fantasy you've been dying to share.

- *Surprise Your Bottom:* Slip a blindfold on him, then let him wait and wonder what's next. Change into a costume, bring out a new toy, or explore every inch of his body with your mouth.

bandannas, or scarves. Blindfolds should be snug, but not too tight. When a blindfold comes off, the person will usually be disoriented and extra-sensitive to light, so keep that in mind.

Taking away a bottom's ability to speak can serve to put someone in a submissive role or quiet an otherwise mouthy individual. Gags come in all shapes and sizes. It's best for beginners to start with a gag made of soft cloth or fabric, like a scarf, bandanna, or even a pair of underwear; these soft gags are the easiest on a bottom's jaw and mouth. More extreme gags, including rubber or plastic "ball gags" (a ball with straps attached to it) and metal horse bits, are inflexible and much more difficult to keep in the mouth; people with jaw or mouth problems should think about avoiding them altogether. When you put a gag in someone's mouth for an extended amount of time, the bottom will inevitably begin to drool—it can't be helped, though this might be a desired side effect if you want to put your bottom in his or her place. Even more important, a gagged bottom cannot use their safeword during a scene; you should both agree on a physical signal to use in place of a safeword.

Putting a hood over someone's head deprives a person of sight and suppresses his or her ability to smell and hear. Hoods can really put a person into an altered state. Because the face and head are completely covered, some people feel a loss of identity. Others have an easier time becoming someone else or slipping into a submissive role when they have a hood on. Make sure the bottom can breathe easily in the hood, and that it isn't too tight anywhere. Hoods are made of nylon, leather, rubber, or a combination of materials and are sold at leather, S/M, and sex-toy stores; you may be tempted to use an oversized winter cap as a hood, but they have no ventilation. You can use a thin cotton pillowcase as long as you don't tie it closed and you make sure the bottom can easily breathe. When a hood comes off, the bottom will be extremely disoriented. Hoods and other forms of sensory deprivation can cause a person to lose sense of balance and time, and otherwise detach from reality; some people describe it as "taking a trip," so be prepared to bring them back down to Earth.

Hot Wax

They softly light a room for lovemaking, they set a mood, and they are romantic, but candles can also be a tantalizing or tortuous BDSM device. Many people enjoy playing with hot wax, dripping it slowly and seductively on someone's body to create a unique sensation. You should always use ordinary white (paraffin) candles for wax play, since colored candles burn much hotter. Never use beeswax candles, which burn at a much higher temperature than ordinary wax candles and will burn the skin.

You can drip hot wax almost anywhere on the body except the neck, face, head, and genitals. Hold a candle several inches away from the body, and gently tip it over. The closer the candle, the hotter the wax will be when it hits the skin. It's best to begin a good distance away from your targeted spot and with a small amount of wax. This is another activity you can (and should) practice on yourself. Try alternating between hot wax and an ice cube to create a wonderfully sexy combination.

Of course, when playing with wax, use your common sense to prevent the candle from coming into contact with highly flammable materials, and be sensible about where you do it, since wax can make a big mess to clean up.

Spanking

Whether it happened to them as a child or not, plenty of adults enjoy a good old-fashioned spanking. A consistent, repeated series of smacks or slaps on someone's flesh, administered with a variety of implements, can be highly erotic and enjoyable. For some, it is a different, very sensual sensation that turns them on; for others, it is the pain—and resulting release of endorphins into the body—that is arousing. In addition to the physical experience, submitting to pain, discipline, or punishment can be highly emotionally charged, which also contributes to the turn-on.

You can spank someone with all sorts of things, including your hand, a slapper, or a paddle. For novices and those looking for a light to moderate sensation, it's best to begin with your own hand. Your hand can help you gauge just how soft or hard you are hitting someone, and is the easiest of tools to master since you've been using it your entire life! Take off rings and bracelets before you spank anyone; they can distract and cause injury. Pick a fleshy area of the body to spank—the most popular, and my personal favorite (surprise, surprise) is the ass. Get your bottom in a comfortable position—for example, lying over your lap, on all fours, or bent over the bed or a table.

Talk to your bottom, tell him or her what you're about to do. Perhaps say why you're giving the spanking if it's part of the scene ("You've been very naughty . . ." "This is because you forgot to thank me for untying you . . ."). If you haven't yet done any foreplay or other touching, before you start spanking, it's a good idea to get the bottom going. The more aroused he or she is, the more enjoyable the spanking will be for both of you. So, lick her pussy a little, stroke his cock, talk dirty to her, suck on his nipples, do whatever it is you know will get your bottom nice and turned on.

Begin by stroking and kneading the butt cheeks. Rubbing them firmly (but not too hard) will help to warm the skin and prepare it for the spanking; plus it will turn your partner on and tempt him or her with what's to come. Slightly cup your hand with the fingers together. Start out very lightly, just tapping the fullest part of the ass; make sure you avoid hitting the tailbone. After this very light spank, gently massage the area you just hit. Begin alternating sides with a light spank, followed by a massage. Keep your hand as close to the ass as possible; the farther away you bring your hand, the less control you have over hitting the exact spot you are aiming for and the more likely you will hit it too hard. You may want to spank with one hand and use the other one to play with her clit or his cock. Genital stimulation will help relax the bottom and make the spanking feel more sensual. Keep it relatively light in the beginning, and don't spank your bottom more than one or two dozen times. You can always have a heavier, longer spanking later. If you're going to spank

Spanking Tricks

- *Something Different:* Alternate the sting of a smack of your hand with a different, gentler sensation like a fur mitt, a textured glove, or a feather. Or try giving a spanking with a leather glove on.

- *Add a Buzz:* Once you've put her over your knee for a spanking, place a vibrator between her legs. With each spank, she'll press against it and get a buzz between her legs. Or give her a dildo to rub against as you smack her ass, and tell her to think about your cock while she's being spanked.

- *Make It Count:* Have the bottom count each smack, it will help him focus on the spanking and anticipate the next lick to come. You can also have him repeat a phrase like, "Please, Mistress, may I have another?" If he forgets to say it or miscounts, you can start back at one.

- *Cool Off:* To create a combination of hot and cold, after a particularly hard spanking or in between two mild sets, rub an ice cube over his ass, making sure to let some water drip between his cheeks.

- *Grooming Tools:* There are a variety of brushes made for grooming horses (found at tack stores), which can be used on the ass to create unique tactile feelings. Rub or "brush" the cheeks with them, or, for a heavier feeling, you can actually spank with some of them. They also leave very interesting marks on the skin.

someone and then do something else to their ass (flog it, cane it, or drip hot wax on it, for example), keep in mind that the skin is now much more sensitive.

When you're ready to try different spanking tools, check your own home for useful equipment like a wooden spoon, spatula, or hairbrush. Or you may want to invest in a toy called a slapper (two pieces of leather sewn together at one end) or a paddle. Some paddles are leather on one side and soft faux fur on the other, so you can alternate between a whack and a gentle caress. There are also paddles made of rubber or wood, which deliver a much stronger, harder smack than their leather counterparts. Because slappers and paddles can be made of a variety of materials, it is important to know your tools before you start wielding them on another person. Most of them can produce a light sensation or a heavy, painful one depending on how much force is behind it. The important thing is to be very familiar with the implement, what different kinds of sensations it is capable of delivering as well as the pain it may inflict. Test out your spanking tools on yourself—if you are flexible enough, you can try hitting your own butt, or you can experiment on your inner thigh.

Caning

Canes used for BDSM play are not the hooked sticks that people walk with, but long, thin rods used for discipline. Think English governess. Canes can be made of rattan, Lucite, or even plastic, and they are about three feet long. Don't be fooled by their thin (many are the thickness of a pen), seemingly innocuous appearance—canes can be very dangerous. These tools may look innocent, but canes can really hurt, *very* easily mark the skin, and even draw blood.

Because it does not require a lot of strength to wield a cane well, they are especially easy for women to use. You don't need to have well-developed muscles and upper-body strength to create some serious pain; in fact, a flick of the wrist is all it takes to deliver a stinging stroke. Practice your caning skills on a pillow to perfect your aim; trying it out on yourself is also wise so you can get a sense of how it feels, and how much force to put behind a blow. Like spanking and paddling, you should massage the area before actually hitting it. Caning should start out lightly, giving the bottom plenty of time between strokes to recover, relax, and breathe.

Because of its flexibility and design, a cane can inflict injury without very much effort on the part of its user. Your bottom should probably have a significant taste for pain if you're going to be playing with canes. The firm stroke of a cane creates a very different sensation than paddles, hands, or whips: it is a sharp, biting, almost burning sensation that one feels at the site of the smack and then, seconds later, spreads from the site. For the most part, you should only cane a person's ass and thighs. Canes are not for the faint-hearted and are definitely an acquired taste!

Flogging

Being struck gently, sensually, or with plenty of force by a flogger can be a mesmerizing experience, a painful one, or a little bit of both. Floggers are whips that have a handle and multiple tails (anywhere from twenty to fifty) made of a variety of materials, most often animal hides. Floggers are different than whips called cats or cat-o'-nine-tails, which have braided or more dense tails and fewer of them. A long, cordlike whip that looks like a snake is a single-tail whip, not a flogger.

Don't make the mistake of selecting a flogger just because it looks pretty. Well-crafted floggers are beautiful and come in magnificent colors and designs, but you want the right tool for the job, not a piece of art. For example, suede and deerskin floggers produce a sensual, warm, light thud and are great for beginners, whereas the leather of a bullhide flogger has more density, is much heavier, and has quite a bite. Besides leather, there are also floggers made of rubber. With prices ranging from sixty-five to three hundred dollars and beyond, a flogger is a serious investment as far as toys go, and the workmanship def-

Flogging Techniques

Figure Eight: Bend your elbow and begin "drawing" figure eights using your wrist and forearm to move the flogger. When you get the hang of it, move toward your practice target and note where the ends of the tails strike.

Horizontal: Like it sounds, this is a horizontal stroke of the flogger. Swing the flogger back and forth in front of you. Use your wrist and forearm, and be careful not to throw your whole body into it. Again, see where the tails land, and that will help you to aim them where you want them.

Vertical: This is a common method you'll see often in demonstrations and videos. Throw the whip over one shoulder and propel it forward with your wrist and forearm. It's easy to hit the shoulders and neck, instead of the meaty area of the back, with this method; here is where the towel-around-the-neck comes in handy for beginners.

initely varies. I recommend that you go to a leather store with experienced, knowledgeable salespeople who can answer your questions reliably. Or better yet, go to a local leather flea market where you can often talk to the whipmakers themselves; tell them what kind of sensation you're looking for, and they'll tell you what hides best suit you.

It is important for you to learn how to flog someone properly before you incorporate flogging into a scene. I absolutely recommend that you go to a workshop on flogging or ask an experienced player to give you a personal tutorial. Local BDSM organizations and stores often sponsor classes by some of the leading practitioners and teachers in the BDSM community. It also helps to watch flogging scenes, whether in a video or at a BDSM club or demonstration. There are some wonderful chapters on flogging in BDSM how-to guides—most notably *Screw the Roses, Send Me the Thorns*—but nothing beats a hands-on approach to this kind of learning. While you are still getting a grip, so to speak, on flogging, it's a good idea to practice your aim, timing, and technique on an inanimate object like a pillow or a large stuffed animal.

Before you've graduated to a real live person, you may want to try having someone else flog you so you can see what it feels like; one of the best ways to learn about doing BDSM as a top is to do it first as a bottom. The most important thing to know about flogging (and any kind of smacking) is that you should only hit the fleshy parts of the body. Most people enjoy being hit on their backs, asses, and thighs. You should avoid all bony areas, joints, and organs, including the head, neck, spine, knees, shins, ankles, elbows, shoulder blades, kidneys, stomach, and genitals. Like anything else new, it takes lots of practice before you can master it. When I started flogging bottoms, I often put a towel around their necks to protect them from my novice aim, which often went off course. It's crucial that a flogging be well paced, with plenty of warm-up, building up to more and more.

Once you've practiced your aim on a pillow and have a willing bottom in front you, take your time. Hold the flogger in your hand and get used to the weight of it. Drape the tails across your bottom's back, dragging them across the body to create a sensual feeling. Massage the area you are going to flog—probably the back and the ass—and slap or spank it lightly to ready it for the whip. There are several ways to throw a flogger, so you should see what works best for you. I like to step back from the person and throw the whip several times without hitting just to warm up. If you have one flogger, make the most of it. Start out using it very lightly, then gradually increase how hard you hit. Tops who own several floggers like to warm up with the softer, lighter ones, then graduate to heavier ones.

It's important to pay attention to your bottom's verbal and non-verbal cues during a flogging. Encourage your partner to talk to you and tell you how it feels, so you can gauge his or her pain tolerance. Let the bottom's feedback guide how you proceed. After several lashes of the whip, approach your partner, massage the areas on her body you've hit, talk to her, reassure her, commend her for her strength and perseverance. You may want to build up to a heavier flogger, then switch back to a lighter one to give her a rest. Also pay attention to her body and how it responds to the whip. Many people flinch slightly, but if you see a more extreme flinch, you are probably hitting too hard. Skilled flogging takes a lot of practice—don't expect to master it the first time around.

Nipple (and Other) Clamps

Whether it was during a childhood romp or at an especially intense moment during sex, we have all learned what it feels like to be pinched. Some folks like to be pinched in specific sweet spots, and a pinch will heighten sexual arousal. Others like to pinch certain areas of the body—especially the nipples, chest, inner thighs, and upper arms—for extended periods of time with implements other than fingers. You can use clothespins, various kinds of clips (like those sold at office-supply stores), or hair clips. There are also a wide variety of nipple clamps available at leather, S/M, and sex-toy stores. When you put a clamp on a part of the body, you cut off the circulation to that area. It definitely hurts (to varying degrees) when you put any kind of a clamp on. But here's the real trick: it feels a hell of a lot worse when the clamp comes off. The blood quickly rushes back to the area in a big burst, and bang, your brain registers pain! The turn-on comes with the release of endorphins from the pain, and from the endurance: how much you can take and how long you can take it. If clamps are tight and left on for a while, they can also leave very unique marks.

Nipple clamps (which are two clamps attached with a chain)

come in a wide variety of styles and strengths, and as their name suggests, are most often used on men's and women's nipples. There are dozens of different varieties and styles to choose from, but a good starter set of clamps are the kind you can adjust, often called "tweezer style." The problem with clothespins, binder clips, and many kinds of nipple clamps is that you can't change the severity of the clamping mechanism, so they have only one clamping strength. With adjustable clamps, you can start out with the loosest clamping and work your way up to a tighter and more severe pinch.

In addition to nipples, look for fleshy areas that you can grab between your fingers—above the breasts, on the back, along the inner thighs, for example. You should definitely work your way up in terms of how much time you leave clamps on in any one area. Bottoms should always tell a top if the pain is intolerable, if it's pinching too much or in a way that doesn't feel good. Never leave any clamp on for more than fifteen minutes.

In the beginning, try putting on just a few strategically placed clothespins and see what feels best to the bottom. Many people like to clamp the area, then a minute later jiggle the clothespins for an added sensation. Leave them on for only a few minutes, then take them off. Remember, the sensation increases tenfold as they come off and the blood rushes back to the area. Experiment with different ways of removing the clothespins: gently squeeze the end, releasing the flesh in the nicest way; or if you want to test your bottom, tug at the pin, let it slide off the skin about halfway, then squeeze the end and release it all the way. You might even rip the clothespin off quickly and mercilessly for a sadistic gesture your bottom won't soon forget.

If you want to start out playing with his or her nipples, invest in the tweezer clamps or any kind of adjustable clamps, so you have a range of options. Again, clothespins may be too tight on nipples and leave you no way to adjust the intensity. If the feeling is too intense when you first put them on, try slipping more of the nipple into the clamp, which should lessen the pinch or decrease the clamping strength. The chain between the pair of clamps is a great way to continue to tease the nipples once the clamps are on—tug on the chain gently, and see how hard you can pull on it. When the clamps are ready to come off, you've got the same options I described for the clothespins, depending on your mood, of course.

Water Sports

"Golden showers" and "water sports" are terms coined by the BDSM community to describe taking pleasure in pee. Golden showerers fetishize the feel, the smell, the taste of piss; they enjoy the erotics of pissing on themselves or on others, or being pissed on. It makes sense that some people into power play would also be into piss: a top can assert dominance by peeing on a bottom, and being pissed on can be the ultimate act of submission. Yet, although golden showers were once associated exclusively with BDSM, it is an activity that is gaining more popularity, acceptance, and practice among nonkinky folks. After all, it can feel really good, and it is another bodily fluid we can share with our lovers.

So what's so sexy about pee? Well, for one thing, a shot of warm liquid all over your body can feel really good, especially if that fluid comes from your lover's body. Many people's fantasies involve the forbiddenness of doing something together that's meant to happen only in private, and the naughtiness of playing with piss can be a big turn-on. They can combine golden showers as part of dominant and submissive role-playing. If you're thinking of experimenting with water sports, a good place to start is the shower—it's steamy, sexy, and the cleanup is automatic!

You may be wondering about the safety of piss play. Contrary to popular belief, urine isn't sterile, but it is very clean as far as bodily fluids go, even cleaner than spit. Peeing on someone or in someone's mouth is pretty low risk. Being peed on or in can be safe, with a few exceptions. Hepatitis B, cytomegalovirus (CMV), the genital herpes virus, chlamydia, and gonorrhea may be present in the urine of a person infected with any of these diseases and can be transmitted through broken skin or a mucous membrane. Swallowing urine that is infected with CMV, chlamydia, and gonorrhea could theoretically lead to infection. There is no research on HIV being transmitted through urine; however, it is possible if there is blood in the urine. Whether water sports are part of your BDSM play or an activity unto itself, be sure you think about cleanup before you start. It's warm, it's wet, but who wants to sleep on a urine-soaked bed?

Psychological Play

Some people who do BDSM don't eroticize pain, never pick up an inflicting instrument, and after scenes, never have a scratch or a bruise. After all this talk of different sensations and playing with pain, how is that possible? Lots of BDSM people are more interested in playing with the mind than the body. Psychological play can be as intense, painful, and exhilarating as any physical play.

There is a whole range of psychological play, and much of it I already discussed in the fantasy and role-playing chapter. People who do BDSM may play some of the same scenarios—mistress/slave, kidnapper/captive, doctor/patient, teacher/student, and others—but they usually take it up a notch by adding other elements of BDSM to role-playing. Some people like to enact erotic dramas that are taboo in our society: parental roles, like mommy or daddy and child; age play, including infantilism, in which people act like babies; or animal play, like a trainer and a horse or an owner and a puppy. Some people also like to play with gender, and embody a gender different from their own.

As part of a scene, some people may crave verbal discipline

or abuse, humiliation, public humiliation, interrogation, punishment, or other seemingly negative scenarios. Why would someone want to do such a thing? Under normal circumstances, no one takes pleasure in being yelled at, humiliated, taunted, criticized, or punished. However, as part of an erotic BDSM scene, the drama, tension, and release that comes from such an exchange—between two people who actually care for each other and have negotiated beforehand—can be cathartic and pleasurable.

Advanced Play

In addition to the practices I've reviewed, there is plenty more to BDSM. If you've found that you enjoy pain and sensations, you may want to try single-tail whipping, cutting, play piercing, or electricity play. If hot wax appeals to you, other hot stuff includes burning, branding, and fire play. You can take bondage one step further with suspension bondage, and sensory deprivation to the next level with breath-control play (including choking). Some people like their genitals played with in a more extreme way, which is called genitorture or genital play. I consider these activities BDSM 201 and up. They require more skill and can be potentially more risky and dangerous. I encourage you to get more information (a workshop, a book, a video) before you try any of these activities.

What is a fetish and how do I know if I have one? What's a fetish party?

In the fabulous photography book *The Beauty of Fetish,* by Steven Diet Goedde, professional dominant FetishDiva Midori writes: "The catalogue of commonly recognized fetish objects are infinite as the creativity of the human mind. . . . What do all these objects have in common for the vast number of individual fetishists today? The power of potential."[23]

A fetish is an inanimate object or a part of the body that turns you on. In technical (and once pathological) terms, a true fetishist *must* have the fetish in order to be aroused and sexually satisfied at all. The term has lost its psychiatric meaning, and now it is used to describe a desire for a particular object, from the moderate to the obsessive. As a fetishist, you may fixate on or have an overwhelming desire to worship certain parts of a lover's body—you've got an ass fetish, a hair fetish, a foot fetish, etc. Or clothing and accessories could be your turn-on: a shoe fetish, an earring fetish, a seamed-stocking fetish. Maybe there are nonsexual things that become highly erotic to you; there are plenty of folks with food fetishes, car fetishes, or uniform fetishes.

The term *fetish* has also expanded in recent years to cover a wide range of tastes and activities. Leather, latex, PVC, and other sexy, kinky clothes are now often referred to as "fetish-wear." Events or gatherings where people dress up and do BDSM scenes might be called a "fetish party." But at the heart of the term is still the notion of eroticism, and in various contexts, fetish still signifies an intense lust that usually takes the form of some *thing*.

Afterword
A Brief Erotic Manifesto

When it comes right down to it, great sex happens when you connect with your partner, when you trust each other and feel comfortable enough to share your desires, explore your fantasies, and open yourself to try new things. I want to encourage everyone to take such a journey with their sexual partner, and I hope I have given you some tools, techniques, and tricks to enhance your sex life. Many of the kinds of sex discussed in the book were once thought of as "alternative" or on the fringe, but I believe that they are becoming more popular among regular, everyday folks than ever before. Believe me, working at a sex-toy store and teaching sex workshops around the country has convinced me that the girl next door has got a strap-on and her boyfriend bought it for her.

Sex can be fun, relaxing, life-affirming, mind-blowing, spiritual, and physically and emotionally fulfilling. Each one of you will take something different from this book—a refresher course on sexual anatomy, tips on erotic communication, a guide to adding toys to sex, encouragement for exploring new areas of the body through G-spot and anal stimulation, ideas for fantasy role-playing, a new perspective on using erotica, or an introduction to the world of BDSM. Do not feel pressure to learn everything at once or perfect your lovemaking skills in a day. Take it one orgasm at a time.

I began the book talking about desire, a complex, sometimes elusive element that doesn't always make sense. Remember that the best techniques in the world won't get you very far if you aren't willing to follow your heart and your libido. Don't deny what turns you on. Embrace your desires fully. Be honest with yourself and your lover and be as direct as you can. Don't compromise your pleasure. Treat your partner and your intimate relationship with as much love and respect as possible.

Sex is a significant, sacred, and powerful force in our lives. Honor and celebrate it—and your own sexual power.

Notes

1. John Leland, "The Science of Women and Sex," *Newsweek,* May 29, 2000, p. 51.
2. Rebecca Chalker, *The Clitoral Truth: The Secret World at Your Fingertips* (New York: Seven Stories Press, 2000), pp. 32 and 35.
3. William H. Masters and Virginia E. Johnson, *Human Sexual Response* (New York: Random House, 1966).
4. Alice Kahn Ladas, Beverly Whipple, and John D. Perry, *The G Spot and Other Discoveries About Human Sexuality* (New York: Dell, 1983), p. 21.
5. Roselyn Payne Epps and Susan Cobb Stewart, eds., *The American Medical Women's Association Guide to Sexuality* (New York: Dell, 1996), p. 158.
6. Phone interview with San Francisco Sex Information Supervisor, May 1997, and Cathy Winks and Anne Semans, *The New Good Vibrations Guide to Sex* (San Francisco: Cleis Press, 1997), p. 73.
7. "Nonoxynol-9 May Increase Risk of HIV," *Sojourner,* September 2000, p. 9.
8. Ladas, Whipple, and Perry, p. 45.
9. According to research by Milan Zaviacic and Beverly Whipple, female ejaculate was found to contain higher levels of prostatic acid phosphatase (PAP) and higher levels of glucose or fructose than are present in urine. Ejaculate was also found to contain lower levels of urea and creatinine, the primary components of urine. From Cathy Winks, *The Good Vibrations Guide: The G-Spot* (San Francisco: Down There Press, 1998), p. 34.

10. A student of Edwin Belzer, who taught human sexuality at Dalhousie University in Nova Scotia, did her own experiment, which Belzer reported in his research: "After taking Uristed tables [a bladder relaxant drug], which dye urine blue, she inspected the 'wet spots' on her sheet following a number of orgasmic explusions. No color whatsoever was apparent in some samples, and in others only the faintest blue tinge appeared. So she intentionally released some urine on the sheet. This time the color was unmistakably a deeper blue." From Ladas, Whipple, and Perry, p. 70.

11. In a study in Spain (reported at the Thirteenth Annual Congress on Sexology in 1997), physicist-psychologist Francisco Cabello Santamaria and clinical analyst Rico Nesters reported the presence of prostate specific antigen (PSA, a primary chemical in male prostatic emissions) in all ejaculation samples. PSA was not present in preorgasmic urine samples, and was present, but in lower quantity, in 75 percent of postorgasmic urine samples. I find the Santamaria/Nesters study one of the most compelling for several reasons. Like other research, their study indicates that ejaculatory fluid is distinctly different from urine—in this case, because of the presence of PSA. The quantity of PSA was high in the ejaculate of the subjects, which supports the theory that the fluid is similar to fluid produced by the prostate gland. From Chalker, p. 98.

12. Ladas, Whipple, and Perry, pp. 80–81.

13. Chalker raises the idea that testosterone and genetics may play a role: "Although there has yet to be a study of the effect that varying testosterone levels in women (or in men for that matter) may have on the production of prostatic fluid, it would seem that the amount of testosterone a woman has may be a determinant in how much ejaculation a woman produces. All women have some testosterone, and while the amount may be influenced by some lifestyle and environmental factors, genetic inheritance may be the strongest single factor." From Chalker, p. 101.

14. Ladas, Whipple, and Perry, p. 69.

15. Ladas, Whipple, and Perry, p. 84.

16. Winks, p. 37.

17. Ladas, Whipple, and Perry, p. 60.

18. Laurence O'Toole, *Pornocopia: Porn, Sex, Technology, and Desire* (London: Serpent's Tail, 1998), p. 6.

19. O'Toole, p. 6.

20. Andrew Wyke, "Exploiting the Many Markets of Adult," *Adult Video News*, September 2000, p. 34.

21. Tod Hunter, "The Condom Revolution Will Not Be Televised," *Adult Video News*, September 2000, pp. 38–40.
22. Marianne Apostolides, "The Pleasure of the Pain: Why Some People Need S&M," *Psychology Today*, September/October 1999, p. 61.
23. FetishDiva Midori, "Contemplation on Fetish and the Pursuit of Our Objects of Desire," in Steven Diet Goedde, *The Beauty of Fetish* (New York: Edition Stemmle, 1998), p. 131.

Resources

1: Sexual Anatomy and Response

BOOKS:

Becoming Orgasmic: A Sexual and Personal Growth Program for Women, by Julia Heiman and Joseph Lopiccolo (New York: Simon & Schuster, 1998).

The Clitoral Truth: The Secret World at Your Fingertips, by Rebecca Chalker (New York: Seven Stories Press, 2000).

Extended Massive Orgasm, by Steve Bodansky and Vera Bodansky (Alameda, CA: Hunter House Publishers, 2000).

The Multi-Orgasmic Couple: Secrets Every Couple Should Know, by Mantak Chia, Maneewan Chia, Douglas Abrams, and Rachel Carlton Abrams, M.D., (San Francisco: HarperSanFrancisco, 2000).

The Multi-Orgasmic Man: Sexual Secrets Every Man Should Know, by Mantak Chia and Douglas Abrams (San Francisco: HarperSanFrancisco, 1997).

The New Male Sexuality: The Truth About Men, Sex, and Pleasure, by Bernie Zilbergeld (New York: Bantam, 1999).

A New View of a Woman's Body, by Federation of Feminist Women's Health Center (Los Angeles: Feminist Health Press, 1991). Note: This will be listed as "out of print" with booksellers; it is only available directly from the publisher, see www.fwhc.org.

Oral Caress: The Loving Guide to Exciting a Woman: A Comprehensive Illustrated

Manual on the Joyful Art of Cunnilingus, by Robert W. Birch (Columbus: Greyden Press, 1999).

Our Bodies, Ourselves: For The New Century, by Boston Women's Health Collective (New York: Touchstone Books, 1998).

Sex for One: The Joy of Selfloving, by Betty Dodson (New York: Crown Publications, 1996).

VIDEOS:

Celebrating Orgasm, directed by Betty Dodson (Betty Dodson, 1996), 60 minutes.

Fire in the Valley: An Intimate Guide to Female Genital Massage, directed by Joseph Kramer and Annie Sprinkle (EroSpirit Research Institute, 1999), 55 minutes.

Fire on the Mountain: An Intimate Guide to Male Genital Massage, directed by Joseph Kramer (EroSpirit Research Institute, 1993), 45 minutes.

Masturbation Memoirs (Volumes 1–4), directed by Dorrie Allen (House O' Chicks, 1995), 15 minutes.

Selfloving, directed by Betty Dodson (Betty Dodson, 1991), 60 minutes.

Viva La Vulva, directed by Betty Dodson (Betty Dodson, 1998), 51 minutes.

2: Erotic Desire, Sexual Communication, and Safer Sex

BOOKS:

Beyond Viagra: A Commonsense Guide to Building a Healthy Sexual Relationship for Both Men and Women, by Gerald A. Melchiode, M.D., with Bill Sloan (New York: Owl Books, 1999).

The Complete Guide to Safer Sex, by the Institute for the Advanced Study of Human Sexuality, edited by Ted McIlvenna (Ft. Lee, NJ: Barricade Books, 1999).

Could It Be . . . Perimenopause?: How Women 35–50 Can Overcome Forgetfulness, Mood Swings, Insomnia, Weight Gain, Sexual Dysfunction, and Other Telltale Signs of Hormonal Imbalance, by Steve R. Goldstein, M.D., and Laurie Ashner (New York: Little Brown & Co., 2000).

The Erotic Mind: Unlocking the Inner Sources of Sexual Passion and Fulfillment, by Jack Morin (New York: HarperCollins, 1996).

The Fine Art of Erotic Talk: How to Entice, Excite and Enchant Your Lover with Words, by Bonnie Gabriel (New York: Bantam, 1996).

For Women Only: A Revolutionary Guide to Overcoming Sexual Dysfunction and Reclaiming Your Sex Life, by Jennifer Berman, M.D., and Laura Berman, Ph.D. (New York: Henry Holt, 2001).

Full Exposure: Opening Up to Sexual Creativity and Erotic Expression, by Susie Bright (San Francisco: HarperSanFrancisco, 2000).

I'm Not in the Mood: What Every Woman Should Know About Improving Her Libido, by Judith Reichman (New York: Quill/William Morrow and Co., 1999).

The Survivor's Guide to Sex: How to Have a Great Sex Life After Child Sexual Abuse, by Staci Haines (San Francisco: Cleis Press, 2000).

Talk Sexy to the One You Love (And Drive Each Other Wild in Bed), by Barbara Keesling (New York: HarperCollins, 1997).

3: Hand Jobs and Oral Sex

BOOKS:

Guide to Getting It On!, by Paul Joannides (Chicago: Goofy Foot Press, 2000).

How to Be a Great Lover; Girlfriend-to-Girlfriend Totally Explicit Techniques That Will Blow His Mind, by Lou Paget (New York: Broadway Books, 1999).

How to Give Her Absolute Pleasure: Totally Explicit Techniques Every Woman Wants Her Man to Know, by Lou Paget (New York: Broadway Books, 2000).

The New Good Vibrations Guide to Sex, by Cathy Winks and Anne Semans (San Francisco: Cleis Press, 1997).

VIDEOS:

Nina Hartley's Advanced Guide to Oral Sex, directed by Nina Hartley (Adam & Eve, 1998), 86 minutes.

Nina Hartley's Guide to Better Cunnilingus, directed by Nina Hartley (Adam & Eve, 1995), 77 minutes.

Nina Hartley's Guide to Better Fellatio, directed by Nina Hartley (Adam & Eve, 1994), 45 minutes.

4: Sex Tools and Sex Toys

BOOKS:

The Black Book: The Guide for the Erotic Explorer, by Bill Brent (San Francisco: Black Books, 2000).

The Go Ask Alice Book of Answers: A Guide to Good Physical, Sexual, and Emotional Health, by Columbia University's Health Education Program (New York: Owl Books, 1998).

Good Vibrations: The New Guide to Vibrators, by Joani Blank and Ann Whidden (San Francisco: Down There Press, 2000).

Mind Your Body: A Sexual Health and Wellness Guide for Women, by Beth Howard (New York: Griffin, 1998).

The Technology of Orgasm: "Hysteria," the Vibrator, and Women's Sexual Satisfaction, by Rachel Maines (Baltimore: John's Hopkins University Press, 1999).

Hot Pants: Do It Yourself Gynecology and Herbal Remedies, by Isabelle Gauthier and Lisa Vinebaum, 1999. This is a booklet distributed by Bloodsisters c/o Elle Corazon, 176 Bernard West, Montreal, Quebec, H2T 2K2 Canada.

Woman to Woman: A Leading Gynecologist Tells You All You Need to Know About Your Body and Your Health, by Yvonne S. Thornton and Jo Coudert (New York: Penguin USA, 1998).

VIDEOS:

Carol Queen's Great Vibrations, directed by Joani Blank (Blank Tapes Productions, 1995), 55 minutes.

Nina Hartley's Guide to Sex Toys, directed by Nina Hartley (Adam & Eve, 1998), 87 minutes.

SEX TOY MANUFACTURERS/DISTRIBUTORS:

California Exotic Novelties, Inc.
14255 Ramona Avenue
Chino, CA 91710
(800) 7-SWEDISH
www.calexotics.com
Mainstream adult toy company.

Doc Johnson Enterprises
11933 Vose Street
North Hollywood, CA 91605

(800) 423-3650
www.docjohnson.com
Mainstream adult toy company.

Dils for Does
(520) 556-9475
Makers of handmade silicone dildos and plugs.

Innerspace
P.O. Box 56328
Sherman Oaks, CA 91413
(818) 897-4444
www.innerspaceart.com
Makers of clear acrylic dildos and butt plugs.

Knowmind Enterprises Inc.
P.O. Box 8070
Madeira Beach, FL 33738
(727) 580-0551
www.knowmind.com
Makers of Pyrex-quality glass dildos.

Scorpio Novelty Products
5414 Kings Highway, First Floor
Brooklyn, NY 11203
(718) 629-6359
Makers of handmade silicone dildos.

Tantus
2856 Delta Drive
Colorado Springs, CO 80910
(719) 391-4200
Makers of handmade silicone dildos.

Vibratex
P.O. Box 991
Vallejo, CA 94590
(800) 222-3361
www.vibratex.com
Makers and distributors of Japanese vibrators, including dual-action models.

Vixen Creations
1004 Revere Ave. B-49
San Francisco, CA 94124

(415) 822-0403
www.vixencreations.com
Makers of handmade silicone dildos, plugs, and anal beads.

5: G-Spot Stimulation and Female Ejaculation

BOOKS:

The Clitoral Truth: The Secret World at Your Fingertips, by Rebecca Chalker (New York: Seven Stories Press, 2000).

Eve's Secrets: A Revolutionary Perspective on Human Sexuality, by Josephine Lowndes Sevely (New York: Random House, 1987).

The Good Vibrations Guide: The G-Spot, by Cathy Winks (San Francisco: Down There Press, 1998).

The G Spot and Other Discoveries About Human Sexuality, by Alice Kahn Ladas, Beverly Whipple, and John D. Perry (New York: Dell, 1983).

A Hand in the Bush: The Fine Art of Vaginal Fisting, by Deborah Addington (Emeryville, CA: Greenery Press, 1998).

VIDEOS:

The Amazing G-spot and Female Ejaculation (Access Instructional Media, 2000), 89 minutes.

Guide to G-Spot & Male Multiple Orgasm (Sinclair Institute, 1999), 60 minutes.

How to Female Ejaculate, directed by Fanny Fatale (Fatale Video, 1992), 47 minutes.

How to Find Your Goddess Spot, directed by Dorrie Allen (House O' Chicks, 1995), 30 minutes.

The Incredible G-Spot, directed by Laura Corn (Merlin/Park Avenue Publishers, 1995), 73 minutes.

The Magic of Female Ejaculation, directed by Dorrie Allen (House O' Chicks, 1995), 15 minutes.

Secrets of Female Sexual Ecstasy, directed by Dennis Miller (Charles Muir and Caroline Muir, 1996), 80 minutes.

Sluts and Goddesses Workshop, directed by Annie Sprinkle and Maria Beatty (1992), 50 minutes.

Tantric Journey to Female Orgasm, directed by Debi Sundahl (Isis Media, 1998), 75 minutes.

6: Anal Sex for Him and Her

BOOKS:

Anal Pleasure & Health: A Guide for Men and Women, by Jack Morin (San Francisco: Down There Press, 1998).
The Strap-On Book, by A. H. Dion (Emeryville, CA: Greenery Press, 1999).
Trust, the Hand Book: A Guide to the Sensual and Spiritual Art of Handballing, by Bert Herrman (San Francisco: Alamo Square Press, 1991).
The Ultimate Guide to Anal Sex for Women, by Tristan Taormino (San Francisco: Cleis Press, 1997).
The Ultimate Guide to Strap-On Sex: A Complete Resource for Men and Women, by Karlyn Lotney, a.k.a. Fairy Butch (San Francisco: Cleis Press, 2000).

VIDEOS:

Bend Over Boyfriend, directed by Shar Rednour (Fatale Video/S.I.R. Video, 1998), 60 minutes.
Bend Over Boyfriend 2: More Rockin', Less Talkin', directed by Shar Rednour and Jackie Strano (S.I.R. Video, 1999), 80 minutes.
Nina Hartley's Guide to Anal Sex, directed by Nina Hartley (Adam & Eve, 1996), 60 minutes.
Tristan Taormino's Ultimate Guide to Anal Sex for Women, directed by Tristan Taormino, Ernest Greene, and John Stagliano (Evil Angel, 1999), 238 minutes.

7: Fantasy and Role-Playing

BOOKS:

Come Play with Me: Games and Toys for Creative Lovers, by Joan Elizabeth Lloyd (New York: Warner Books, 1994).
The Couples Guide to Erotic Games: Bringing Intimacy and Passion Back Into Sex and Relationships, by Gerald Schoenewolf (Secaucus, NJ: Citadel Press, 1998).
The Ethical Slut: A Guide to Infinite Sexual Possibilities, by Dossie Easton and Catherine A. Liszt (Emeryville, CA: Greenery Press, 1998).
Exhibitionism for the Shy: Show Off, Dress Up, and Talk Hot, by Carol Queen (San Francisco: Down There Press, 1995).
Forbidden Flowers: More Women's Sexual Fantasies, by Nancy Friday (New York: Pocket Books, 1993).

Fantasex: A Book of Erotic Games for the Adult Couple, by Rolf Milonas (New York: Putnam, 1983).

Getting Close: A Lover's Guide to Embracing Fantasy and Heightening Sexual Connection, by Barbara Keesling (New York: HarperCollins, 1999).

His Secret Life: Male Sexual Fantasies, by Bob Berkowitz (New York: Pocket Books, 1998).

Hot Monogamy: Essential Steps to More Passionate, Intimate Lovemaking, by Dr. Patricia Love and Jo Robinson (New York: Plume, 1999).

My Secret Garden: Women's Sexual Fantasies, by Nancy Friday (New York: Pocket Books, 1998).

The New Intimacy: Open-Ended Marriage and Alternative Lifestyles, by Ronald Mazur (New York: toExcel/iUniverse.com, 2000).

Nice Couples Do: How to Turn Your Secret Dreams into Sensational Sex, by Joan Elizabeth Lloyd (New York: Warner Books, 1991).

Polyamory: The New Love Without Limits, by Deborah M. Anapol (San Raphael, CA: Intinet Resource Center, 1997).

Whispered Secrets: The Couple's Guide to Erotic Fantasies, by Iris and Steve Finz (New York: Penguin, 1990).

Women on Top: How Real Life Has Changed Women's Sexual Fantasies, by Nancy Friday (New York: Pocket Books, 1993).

VIDEOS:

Nina Hartley's Guide to Private Dancing, directed by Nina Hartley (Adam & Eve, 1997), 75 minutes.

8: Adding Erotica to Sex

PUBLICATIONS:

Adult Video News (AVN)
Subscription Office
9414 Eton Avenue
Chatsworth, CA 91311
(818) 718-5788
www.avn.com
Leading adult-industry monthly magazine with video reviews, performer profiles, news, and features.

Adam Film World
8060 Melrose Avenue
Los Angeles, CA 90046

(213) 653-8060
Adult-industry magazine with video reviews and other sex-industry features.

Batteries Not Included
130 W. Limestone Street
Yellow Springs, OH 45387
(973) 767-7416
BNI@aol.com
Offbeat newsletter about the adult industry and other sexy stuff.

Spectator Magazine
P.O. Box 1984
Berkeley, CA 94701
(510) 849-1615
www.spectatormag.com
*California's original adult-news magazine covering several aspects of the sex
industry.*

EROTICA BOOKS:

Best American Erotica series, edited by Susie Bright (New York: Touchstone
   Books, 1993–2001).
Best Bisexual Erotica, edited by Bill Brent and Carol Queen (Cambridge,
   MA: Circlet Press/Black Books, 2000).
Best Black Women's Erotica, edited by Blanche Richardson (San Francisco:
   Cleis Press, 2001).
Best Gay Erotica series, edited by Richard Labonte (San Francisco: Cleis
   Press, 1997–).
Best Lesbian Erotica series, edited by Tristan Taormino (San Francisco: Cleis
   Press, 1996–).
Best Women's Erotica series, edited by Marcy Sheiner (San Francisco: Cleis
   Press, 2000–).
Black Feathers: Erotic Dreams, by Cecilia Tan (New York: HarperCollins,
   1998).
The Erotic Edge: 22 Erotic Stories for Couples, edited by Lonnie Garfield Bar-
   bach (New York: Plume, 1996).
Herotica: A Collection of Women's Erotic Fiction, tenth-anniversary edition,
   edited by Susie Bright (Down There Press/Plume, 1998).
Herotica 2: A Collection of Women's Erotic Fiction, edited by Susie Bright and
   Joani Blank (Down There Press/Plume, 1992).
Herotica 3: A Collection of Women's Erotic Fiction, edited by Susie Bright
   (Down There Press/Plume, 1994).

Herotica 4, 5, 6, and *7,* edited by Marcy Sheiner (Down There Press/ Plume, 1996, 1998, 1999, 2001).

The Leatherdaddy and the Femme, by Carol Queen (San Francisco: Cleis Press, 1998).

Macho Sluts, by Pat Califia (Los Angeles: Alyson Publications, 1989).

Melting Point, by Pat Califia (Los Angeles: Alyson Publications, 1996).

BOOKS ABOUT EROTICA AND ADULT VIDEOS:

The Couple's Guide to the Best Erotic Videos, by Steve and Elizabeth Brent (New York: St. Martin's Press, 1997).

The Edge of the Bed: How Dirty Pictures Changed My Life, by Lisa Palac (New York: Little, Brown & Company, 1998).

The Good Vibrations Guide: Adult Videos, by Cathy Winks (San Francisco: Down There Press, 1998).

Tales from the Clit: A Female Experience of Pornography, by Cherie Matrix (San Francisco: AK Press Distribution, 1996).

The Wise Woman's Guide to Erotic Videos: 300 Sexy Videos for Every Woman and Her Lover, by Angela Cohen and Sarah Gardner Fox (New York: Broadway Books, 1997).

The X-Rated Videotape Guide XIII, by Patrick Riley (Amherst, NY: Prometheus Books, 1999).

ADULT VIDEO PRODUCTION COMPANIES:

Adam & Eve
302 Meadowlands Drive
Hillsborough, NC 27278
(800) 274-0333
www.adameve.com
Mainstream producers/distributors of adult features, including couples-oriented videos, Candida Royalle's Femme videos, and Nina Hartley's how-to videos.

Betty Dodson Productions
P.O. Box 1933
Murray Hill Station
New York, NY 10156
(212) 679-4240
www.bettydodson.com
Producer/distributor of all Betty Dodson videos.

Bizarre Video
20 Jay Street, 5th Floor

Brooklyn, NY 11201
(718) 802-1251
www.bizarrevideo.com
Producers/distributors of mainstream BDSM and fetish videos, including many of director Ernest Greene's videos.

Bleu Productions
P.O. Box 20280
New York, NY 10011
(888) 375-2464
www.bleuproductions.com
Producers of artsy lesbian BDSM and fetish videos.

Blue Door Videos
ETP, Inc.
P.O. Box 64378
Sunnyvale, CA 94089
www.bluedoor.com
Rent or buy adult videos and DVDs on the Internet!

EroSpirit Research Institute
P.O. Box 3893
Oakland, CA 94609
(510) 428-9063
www.erospirit.org
Producer/distributor of erotic videos by Joseph Kramer, Annie Sprinkle, and others.

Evil Angel
14141 Covello Street, Unit 8-C
Van Nuys, CA 91405
(800) 442-6435
www.evilangel.com
Producer/distributor of videos by Gregory Dark, John Leslie, John Stagliano, and others.

Fatale Video
1537 4th Street, #193
San Raphael, CA 94901
(888) 5-FATALE
www.other-rooms.com/fatale.html
Lesbian-produced lesbian videos.

Femme Productions
P.O. Box 268

New York, NY 10012
(800) 456-LOVE
www.royalle.com
Candida Royalle's adult videos from a woman's perspective.

House O' Chicks
2215-R Market Street #813
San Francisco, CA 94114
(415) 861-9849
www.houseochicks.com
Producers/distributors of feminist, alternative short erotic videos.

Isis Media
369 Montezuma, Suite 112
Santa Fe, NM 87501
(505) 988-1909
www.isismedia.org
Producer of tantric sex and other erotic videos.

Jill Kelly Productions
P.O. Box 691447
9127 Thrasher Avenue
Los Angeles, CA 90069
(866) 550-3934
www.jillkellyproductions.com
Porn star Jill Kelly's company, producers and distributors of adult videos.

Libido Films
P.O. Box 146721
Chicago, IL 60614
www.libido.com
Former publishers of Libido *magazine, now producers of couples-oriented videos.*

Metro
9315 Oso Street
Chatsworth, CA 91311
(888) 963-8769
www.metroglobal.com
Mainstream producers/distributors of adult features, including couples-oriented videos.

Shane's World
13659 Victory Blvd. PMB 616
Van Nuys, CA 91401

www.shanesworld.com
Distributed by The Odyssey Group, several video series include Shane's World
and the all-girl Slumber Party.

Sin City
9155 Deering Avenue
Chatsworth, CA 91311
(818) 407-9990
*Mainstream producers/distributors of adult features, including couples-oriented
videos.*

Sinclair Intimacy Institute
101 Conner Drive, Suite 302
Hillsborough, NC 27514
www.intimacyinstitute.com
*Producers of the Better Sex Video Series, couples-oriented instructional videos
produced in cooperation with leading sexuality educators and therapists with
commentary by experts and explicit demonstrations by couples.*

S.I.R. Video
3288 21st Street PMB #94
San Francisco, CA 94110
(415) 978-0891
www.sirvideo.com
Producers of how-to videos and lesbian-produced lesbian porn.

Studio A Entertainment
1625 Stanford Street
Santa Monica, CA 90404
(310) 450-2669
www.andrewblake.com
Producer/distributor of director Andrew Blake's adult videos.

VCA
9650 De Soto Avenue
Chatsworth, CA 91311
(800) 421-2386
www.vcaexposed.com
*Mainstream producers/distributors of adult features, including couples-oriented
videos.*

Video Team
15753 Stagg Street
Van Nuys, CA 91406

(818) 997-3311

www.afro-centric.com

Mainstream producers/distributors of adult videos, including the Afro-Centric line focused on people of color.

Vivid Film & Video

15127 Califa Street

Van Nuys, CA 91411

(800) 822-8339

www.vividvideo.com

Mainstream producers/distributors of adult features, including couples-oriented videos.

Wicked Pictures

9040 Eton Avenue

Canoga Park, CA 91304

(818) 349-3593

www.wickedweb.com

Mainstream producers/distributors of adult features, including couples-oriented videos.

Xplor Media/Homegrown Video

P.O. Box 420820

San Diego, CA 92142

(858) 541-0280

www.homegrownvideo.com

Producers/distributors of amateur adult videos.

9: Exploring BDSM

BOOKS:

The Bottoming Book: How to Get Terrible Things Done to You by Wonderful People, by Dossie Easton and Catherine A. Liszt (Emeryville, CA: Greenery Press, 1998).

Come Hither: A Commonsense Guide to Kinky Sex, by Gloria G. Brame (New York: Fireside, 2000).

The Compleat Spanker, by Lady Green (Emeryville, CA: Greenery Press, 1998).

Different Loving: The World of Sexual Dominance and Submission, by Gloria Brame, Will Brame, and Jon Jacobs (New York: Villard, 1996).

Flogging, by Joseph W. Bean (Emeryville, CA: Greenery Press, 2000).

Jay Wiseman's Erotic Bondage Handbook, by Jay Wiseman (Emeryville, CA: Greenery Press, 2000).

Learning the Ropes: A Basic Guide to Safe and Fun S/M Lovemaking, by Race Bannon (San Francisco: Daedelus Press, 1993).

Leathersex: A Guide for the Curious Outsider and the Serious Player, by Joseph Bean (San Francisco: Daedalus Publishing Co., 1997).

The Mistress Manual: The Good Girl's Guide to Female Dominance, by Lorelei (Emeryville, CA: Greenery Press, 2000).

Screw the Roses, Send Me the Thorns: The Romance and Sexual Sorcery of Sado-masochism, by Philip Miller and Molly Devon (Fairfield, CT: Mystic Rose Books, 1996).

The Sexually Dominant Woman: A Workbook for Nervous Beginners, by Lady Green (Emeryville, CA: Greenery Press, 1998).

SM 101: A Realistic Introduction, by Jay Wiseman (Emeryville, CA: Greenery Press, 1998).

The Topping Book: Or, Getting Good at Being Bad, by Dossie Easton and Catherine A. Liszt (Emeryville, CA: Greenery Press, 1998).

Training with Miss Abernathy: A Workbook for Erotic Slaves and Their Owners, by Christina Abernathy (Emeryville, CA: Greenery Press, 1998).

When Someone You Love Is Kinky, by Dossie Easton and Catherine A. Liszt (Emeryville, CA: Greenery Press, 2000).

VIDEOS:

Learning the Ropes series, directed by Frank Zee and Ona Zee (Ona Zee Productions), 85 minutes each.

BDSM RETAILERS:

Adam and Gillian's Sensual Whips & Toys
c/o Utopian Network
P.O. Box 1146
New York, NY 10156
(631) 842-1711
www.aswgt.com
Whips, paddles, straps, canes, and other BDSM equipment.

Aslan Leather
Box 102, Stn. B
Toronto, Ontario M5T 2T3, Canada

(416) 306-0462
www.aslanleather.com
Women-owned and -run maker of leather and vinyl dildo harnesses and BDSM accoutrements.

Dressing for Pleasure
590 Valley Road
Upper Montclair, NJ 07043
www.dfp.com
(888) 746-4202
Retail store and mail-order catalog of BDSM toys and clothing, specializing in fetishwear.

Heartwood Whips of Passion
P.O. Box 490
Herndon, VA 20172
(703) 834-0757
www.heartwoodwhips.com
Makers of leather and rubber floggers and whips.

Lashes by Sarah
(866) 333-7867
www.lashesbysarah.com
Makers of leather and rubber floggers and whips.

Leather Man
111 Christopher Street
New York, NY 10014
(212) 243-5339
www.theleatherman-nyc.com
Retail store of leather clothing, BDSM equipment, and sex toys.

Purple Passion
242 West 16th Street
New York, NY 10011
(212) 807-0486
www.purplepassion.com
Retail store of fetishwear, BDSM equipment, and sex toys.

Mr. S Leathers/Fetters
310 7th Avenue
San Francisco, CA 94103
(415) 863-7764
World's largest leather and latex manufacturer and retailer.

The Stockroom/JT's
2140 Hyperion Avenue
Los Angeles, CA 90027
(800) 755-TOYS
www.stockroom.com
Retail and mail-order BDSM and bondage gear.

Stormy Leather
1158 Howard Street
San Francisco, CA 94103
(800) 486-9650
www.stormyleather.com
Retailer and producer of leather and latex fetishwear, dildo harnesses, and sex toys.

Other Books

The Art of Sexual Ecstasy: The Path of Sacred Sexuality for Western Lovers, by Margo Anand (New York: Putnam, 1991).

The Art of Tantric Sex: Ancient Techniques and Rituals That Enhance Sexual Pleasure, by Nitya Lacroix (New York: DK Publishing, 1997).

Bi Any Other Name: Bisexual People Speak Out, by Loraine Hutchins and Lani Kaahumanu (Los Angeles: Alyson Publications, 1991).

Big Big Love: A Sourcebook on Sex for People of Size and Those Who Love Them, by Hanne Blank (Emeryville, CA: Greenery Press, 2000).

The Essential Tantra: A Modern Guide to Sacred Sexuality, by Kenneth Ray Stubbs (New York: Putnam, 2000).

The Hormone of Desire: The Truth About Testosterone, Sexuality and Menopause, by Susan Rako, M.D. (New York: Three Rivers Press, 1999).

The Red Thread of Passion: Spirituality and the Paradox of Sex, by David Guy (Boston: Shambhala Publications, 1999).

Tantra: The Art of Conscious Loving, by Charles and Caroline Muir (San Francisco: Mercury House, 1990).

Other Videos

Annie Sprinkle's Herstory of Porn, directed by Annie Sprinkle (EroSpirit Research Institute, 1999), 69 minutes.

Nina Hartley's Making Love to Men, directed by Nina Hartley (Adam & Eve, 2000), 140 minutes.

Nina Hartley's Making Love to Women, directed by Nina Hartley (Adam & Eve, 2000), 140 minutes.

Sex-Toy Stores and Catalogs

Adam and Eve
P.O. Box 200
Carrboro, NC 27510
(919) 644-1212
(800) 274-0333
www.adameve.com
Mainstream mail-order catalog of toys, videos, lingerie.

A Woman's Touch
600 Williamson Street
Madison, WI 53703
(608) 250-1928
www.a-womans-touch.com
Woman-owned and -run retail store of toys, books, and safer sex supplies.

Blowfish
2261 Market Street #284
San Francisco, CA 94114
(415) 252-4340
(800) 325-2569
www.blowfish.com
Mail-order catalog of toys, books, and videos.

Cetra Latex-Free Supplies
(888) LATEX-NO
www.latexfree.com
Supplier of nitrile, vinyl, and polyurethane safer sex materials.

Come Again Erotic Emporium
353 E. 53rd Street
New York, NY 10022
(212) 308-9394
Store and mail-order catalog of toys, books, and lingerie.

Come As You Are
701 Queen Street West
Toronto, Ontario M6J 1E6, Canada
(877) 858-3160
www.comeasyouare.com
Worker-owned cooperative retail store and mail-order catalog of books, toys, and videos; also offers classes and workshops.

Crimson Phoenix
1876 SW 5th Avenue
Portland, OR 97201
(503) 228-0129
www.crimsonphoenix.org
Retail store of books, toys, and novelties.

Eve's Garden
119 W. 57th Street #420
New York, NY 10019-2383
(212) 757-8651
(800) 848-3837
www.evesgarden.com
Woman-owned and -run feminist store and catalog of toys, books, and videos.

Fetishes Boutique
704 S. 5th Street
Philadelphia, PA 19147
(215) 829-4986
www.fetishesboutique.com
Retail store of sex toys, BDSM equipment, and fetishwear.

Forbidden Fruit
108 East North Loop Blvd.
Austin, TX 78751
(800) 315-2029
www.forbiddenfruit.com
Woman-owned and run retail store of toys, books, and videos.

Good for Her
171 Harbord Street
Toronto, Ontario M5S 1H5, Canada
(877) 588-0900
www.goodforher.com
Woman-owned and -run retail store and mail-order catalog of books, toys, and videos; also offers classes and workshops.

Good Vibrations
1210 Valencia Street
San Francisco, CA 94110
(415) 974-8980 SF store
(510) 841-8987 Berkeley store
(415) 974-8990 mail order

www.goodvibes.com
Worker-owned cooperative retail stores and mail-order catalog of books, toys, and videos; also offers classes and workshops.

Grand Opening!
318 Harvard Street #32
Arcade Building, Coolidge Corner
Brookline, MA 02146
(617) 731-2626
www.grandopening.com
Woman-owned and -run retail store and mail-order catalog of books, toys, and videos; also offers classes and workshops.

Intimacies
28 Center Street
Northampton, MA 01060
(413) 582-0709
www.intimaciesonline.com
Woman-owned and -run retail store of books, toys, and videos; also offers classes and workshops.

It's My Pleasure
3106 NE 64th
Portland, OR 97213
(503) 280-8080
Women-focused retail store of books, toys, and videos.

Loveseason
4001 198th Street SW #7
Lynnwood, WA 98036
(800) 500-8843
Retail store and mail-order catalog of toys, videos, books, and lingerie.

Miko Exoticwear
653 North Main St.
Providence, RI 02904
(401) 421-6646
www.mikoexoticwear.com
Retail and wholesale toys, books, and fetishwear.

Pleasure Chest
7733 Santa Monica Blvd.
West Hollywood, CA 90046
(213) 650-1022 store

(800) 75-DILDO mail order
www.thepleasurechest.com
Retail store and catalog of toys and clothing.

Toys in Babeland
707 E. Pike Street
Seattle, WA 98122
(206) 328-2914 store
(800) 658-9119 mail order
94 Rivington Street
New York, NY 10002
(212) 375-1701
www.babeland.com
Woman-owned and -run retail stores and mail-order catalog of books, toys, and videos; also offers classes and workshops.

WomynsWare
896 Commercial Drive
Vancouver, BC V5L 3Y5, Canada
(604) 254-2543
www.womynsware.com
Woman-owned and -run retail store and mail-order catalog of books, toys, and videos.

Xandria Collection
165 Valley Drive
Brisbane, CA 94005
(415) 468-3812
(800) 242-2823
www.xandria.com
Mainstream mail-order catalog of toys, videos, and lingerie.

Hot Lines

Centers for Disease Control National AIDS Clearinghouse
(800) 342-AIDS
www.cdcnac.com

National AIDS Hotline
(800) 342-2437

National STD Hotline
(800) 227-8922

Planned Parenthood
(800) 230-PLAN
www.ppfa.org

San Francisco Sex Information
(415) 989-7374
www.sfsi.org

Web Sites

AltSex
www.altsex.org
BDSM information.

Erotica Reader's Association
www.erotica-readers.com
Erotic fiction, reviews, and links; one of the best erotica sources on the web.

Jane's Net Sex Guide
www.janesguide.com
Sex-related Web site reviews.

Sexuality Information and Education Council of the U.S.
www.siecus.org
Sex education information.

Society for Human Sexuality
www.sexuality.org
Extensive library and resources on sexuality.

Workshops

Many of the stores listed above offer workshops. Contact individual locations for details.

Betty Dodson
P.O. Box 1933
Murray Hill Station
New York, NY 10156
(212) 679-4240
www.bettydodson.com
Conducts one-on-one masturbation coaching sessions in New York City area.

Body Electric School
6527-A Telegraph Avenue
Oakland, CA 94609
(510) 653-1594
www.bodyelectric.org
San Francisco–area workshops in sexual healing and erotic spirituality, including tantra and Taoist principles.

The Fairy Butch Dynasty
www.fairybutch.com
San Francisco–area workshops taught by Good Vibrations veteran and sex-advice columnist Karlyn Lotney.

FetishDiva Midori
P.O. Box 330064
San Francisco, CA 94133
(415) 584-5200
www.fetishdiva.com
Offers workshops as well as one-on-one sessions in a variety of BDSM activities.

QSM
P.O. Box 880154
San Francisco, CA 94188
(415) 550-7776
www.qualitysm.com
San Francisco–area BDSM workshops taught by various leading experts.

Vulva University
c/o House O' Chicks
2215-R Market Street #813
San Francisco, CA 94114
(415) 861-9849
www.houseochicks.com
Feminist and lesbian sexuality online workshops.

About the Author

Tristan Taormino is the author of *The Ultimate Guide to Anal Sex for Women* (Cleis Press), winner of a 1998 Firecracker Award. She is director, producer, and star of the videos *Tristan Taormino's Ultimate Guide to Anal Sex for Women 1* and *2* (Evil Angel Video), based on her book. She is a columnist for *The Village Voice, Taboo,* Penthouse.com, and her own Web site, Puckerup.com. She is editor of *On Our Backs* magazine. She is series editor of *Best Lesbian Erotica* (Cleis Press), and co-editor of *A Girl's Guide to Taking Over the World: Writings from the Girl Zine Revolution* (St. Martin's Press). She has been featured in more than one hundred publications including *Playboy, Penthouse, RedBook, Entertainment Weekly, Details, New York Magazine, Out,* and *Spin.* She has appeared on MTV, HBO's *Real Sex, The Howard Stern Show, Loveline,* and the Discovery Channel/Canada. She teaches sex workshops and lectures on sex nationwide.